Clinical Pathology for the Veterinary Team

Clinical Pathology for the Veterinary Team

Andrew J. Rosenfeld, DVM

Diplomate, American Board of Veterinary Practitioners
Canine and Feline

Sharon M. Dial, DVM

Diplomate, American College of Veterinary Pathologists
Clinical and Anatomic Pathology

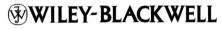

A John Wiley & Sons, Ltd., Publication

Edition first published 2010
© 2010 Blackwell Publishing Ltd.

Blackwell Publishing was acquired by John Wiley & Sons in February 2007. Blackwell's publishing program has been merged with Wiley's global Scientific, Technical, and Medical business to form Wiley-Blackwell.

Editorial office
2121 State Avenue, Ames, Iowa 50014-8300, USA

For details of our global editorial offices, for customer services, and for information about how to apply for permission to reuse the copyright material in this book, please see our website at www.wiley.com/wiley-blackwell.

Library of Congress Cataloging-in-Publication Data

Rosenfeld, Andrew J.
  Clinical pathology for the veterinary team / Andrew J. Rosenfeld, Sharon Dial.
    p. ; cm.
  Includes bibliographical references and index.
    ISBN 978-0-8138-1008-9 (pbk. : alk. paper) 1. Veterinary pathology–Laboratory manuals.
I. Dial, Sharon. II. Title.
    [DNLM: 1. Animal Diseases–pathology–Laboratory Manuals. 2. Clinical Laboratory
Techniques–veterinary–Laboratory Manuals. 3. Pathology, Veterinary–methods–Laboratory Manuals.
SF 772.6 R813c 2010]
    SF772.6.R67 2010
    636.089′607–dc22

                                                                                    2010004690

A catalog record for this book is available from the U.S. Library of Congress.

Set in 10/12pt Sabon by Aptara® Inc., New Delhi, India
Printed in Singapore

1 2010

Dedicated to Lisa, Lauren, and Jillian—who act as my center, my practicality, my imagination, and my world, respectively.

Andrew J. Rosenfeld

Dedicated to the hardworking technicians in veterinary medicine who inspire, challenge, and energize me with every interaction.

Sharon Dial

Contents

Cases – DVD is no longer available

About the Authors

Andrew J. Rosenfeld, DVM, ABVP
Dr. Rosenfeld has been practicing emergency medicine for the last 18 years. His medical interests are in emergency/critical care, ultrasound, internal medicine, and surgery. Dr. Rosenfeld has always had a strong interest in teaching and has been an instructor at Arizona State University and Mesa Community College in Animal Science and Technology. Dr. Rosenfeld is cofounder and head instructor of VTEC, and he has written a training and interactive text for veterinary hospitals called *The Veterinary Medical Team Handbook*, published by Wiley-Blackwell.

Sharon M. Dial, DVM, PhD, Diplomate ACVP (Clinical and Anatomic Pathology)
Dr. Dial received a bachelor's degree in Microbiology from Montana State University. She then received a Doctor of Veterinary Medicine and a Doctorate in Pathology from Colorado State University. Dr. Dial has been both a working pathologist as well as an active instructor at the University of Wisconsin and Louisiana State University. She also has been a clinical pathologist for Animal Diagnostic Lab in Tucson, Arizona, and Antech Diagnostics. Dr. Dial is currently an Associate Research Scientist in the Department of Veterinary Science and Microbiology at the University of Arizona.

Foreword

With new technology, in-hospital clinical diagnostic laboratories are becoming an expected part of every veterinary hospital. Veterinary teams now have the ability to obtain medical data in complete blood count, chemistry, blood gas, lactate, urine, and clotting times in minutes—information that would take 1–2 days to obtain from an outside lab. This allows us to have an excellent medical database quickly and effectively to help evaluate and treat our patients.

However, with this technology comes an added responsibility for our medical team. Team members now must begin to assume the role of the veterinary lab technician. Hospital teams must be able to run quality control on lab equipment and calibrate it as needed. The technical team must be able to handle blood samples and identify potential artifacts. Further, the technical team members must be able to evaluate blood films to identify abnormal cellular pathology that the clinical diagnostics cannot interpret.

Our medical team must be able to train its members in pre-cage theory. This theory states that our hospital team members have an understanding of each patient's disease process, its symptoms, the clinical diagnostics that need to be obtained, and treatment protocols. **They are not expected to be veterinarians,** but no team member should be given the responsibility of monitoring a patient without understanding the disease process affecting the ill animal.

The goal of this book is to help team members understand each clinical diagnostic test of the small animal patient and thus be a more thorough resource to the veterinary team. Each member should be able to monitor patients and communicate concerns to the veterinarian, to discuss these clinical diagnostics with the client, and to understand what further tests and samples may need to be taken when there is a change in clinical pathology.

The DVD at the end of this text is meant to give technical team members the ability to practice the concepts discussed by this book in virtual cases.

Sample Handling and Laboratory Standardization—Developing Standard Operating Procedures

Over the last decade, the availability of hematology and clinical chemistry instrumentation for in-clinic use has increased exponentially. There is a wide choice of instruments being marketed for use in veterinary practices. While the convenience of rapid result turnaround is touted as a primary reason for purchase and use of in-clinic instrumentation, the full impact of their use on technical personnel time or training needs and the full cost of appropriate management of the in-clinic laboratory are usually not well addressed during the decision process. When a veterinary practice decides to provide in-clinic clinical pathology service, it must make the commitment to ensure that the data produced by its in-clinic laboratory is of the same quality as that obtained by reference laboratories. The management of the practice must understand the need for trained personnel, standard operating procedures, and appropriate quality control and quality assurance programs.

The In-House Clinical Laboratory

Once a veterinary practice decides to purchase in-clinic clinical pathology instrumentation, it is the veterinary technician who is given the responsibility to obtain accurate data from the diagnostic samples for clinical management of the patient. This chapter is an introduction to laboratory management. The first aspect of integrating an in-clinic laboratory into the general practice is to identify a location for the laboratory equipment with sufficient workspace that includes space for sample processing, sample/reagent storage, and instrumentation. The area should be convenient to the treatment/surgery areas and examination rooms but out of congested traffic areas. In addition to hematology and clinical chemistry instrumentation, a free-arm centrifuge for spinning down serum and urine samples, a microhematocrit centrifuge, a

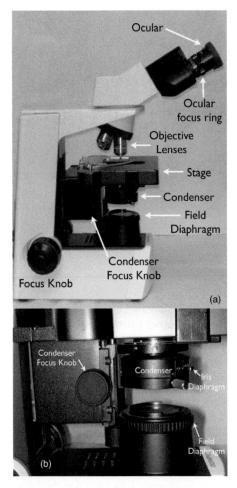

Figure 1.1. Image of a high-quality microscope as part of the in-hospital medical lab equipment.

quality microscope, and a refrigerator with a non–frost-free freezer compartment are needed.

The need for a quality microscope cannot be emphasized enough. The ability to critically examine hematology and cytology specimens depends upon the clear optics of the microscope. Figure 1.1 identifies the components of a compound bright field microscope. The objective lenses of the microscope should be the highest quality affordable. The standard lenses on most light microscopes are 10×, 40×, and 100× oil emersion. The addition of a 20× or a 50× oil emersion lens can facilitate the rapid examination of cytology and hematology samples. Each microscope manufacturer can provide options for magnification and optical correction and should be able to assist in the choice of objectives for the type of clinical use in each practice. Objective lenses differ considerably in cost. It is worth the additional cost for higher-quality lenses that provide a large, flat viewing field. The higher-quality objective will significantly reduce eyestrain experience by the microscopist and improve diagnostic accuracy by providing the best quality image for viewing.

One important note is that the 40× high dry objective requires a coverslipped slide. The optics of this objective are optimized for viewing histopathology slides that are always coverslipped. A simple way to use the 40× objective to view hematology and cytology slides is to use a drop of immersion oil as a coverslip mounting medium. Place a drop of oil on the microscope slide and place a coverslip in top of the oil. This will allow sharp focus of the slide with the 40× objective. It is imperative that the high dry objective does not get immersed in oil. If this inadvertently happens, immediate cleaning with a quality lens cleaner (not xylene) and lens paper is necessary. A good habit is to always rotate the microscope objectives in one direction, from lowest power to highest power. This will keep the microscopist from dragging the 40× objective through oil.

The microscope manufacturer and the individual who is chosen to clean and maintain the scope are great resources for choosing good immersion oil. Immersion oils have been standardized over the years and the most frequently asked question is concerning the viscosity of the oil. High-viscosity oils are often preferred by

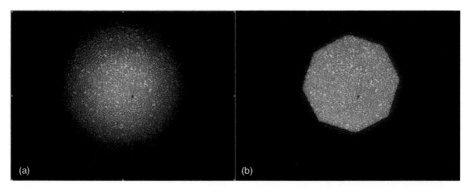

Figure 1.2. **(a)** An out-of-focus field diaphragm with fuzzy edges. **(b)** An in-focus field diaphragm with sharp edges.

microscopists because less oil is required to fill the gap between the slide and the objective lens (high-viscosity oil does not spread out as much as low-viscosity oil) and, when viewing multiple slides, less oil is needed on subsequent slides because the oil clings to the objective when the previous slide is removed. To prevent oil dropping on the next slide before it is needed, the microscopist should develop a habit of switching to the 10× objective before removing one slide and placing a new slide on the stage.

As with all laboratory equipment, maintenance is necessary to keep the microscope working appropriately. A yearly maintenance and cleaning schedule will result in a long and useful life for a good microscope. Microscopy training is essential for all personnel using the microscope. Tasks that should be understood by all microscopists include adjusting the microscope condenser to provide the best illumination (**Köhler illumination**), correct lens cleaning techniques, and bulb replacement. Köhler illumination is the process of adjusting the condenser to produce the best focus of the illumination source. The process is as follows:

1. Place a microscope slide on the stage and focus the image on the slide to 10×.
2. Close the field diaphragm completely.

3. Carefully move the condenser up or down to bring the edges of the field diaphragm into sharp focus (Figure 1.2).
4. Open the field diaphragm to allow complete illumination of the field.

Most good-quality microscopes sold today have an adjustable condenser and are parfocal. **Parfocal** means that if the image is in focus at 10×, there should be little need to focus at the higher magnification objectives. One way to optimize the parfocal lenses is to focus a microscope slide at the higher objective (preferably at 40×) and switch to the 10× objective. If the image is out of focus, use the focus rings of the eyepieces to bring the image back into focus. Once this is done, only fine focus should be needed as the microscopist moves from one objective to the next.

An excellent resource for microscopy tips is the individual that is contracted to maintain the microscope. In addition, there are excellent Internet resources for microscopy. Optimizing microscopy skills will allow veterinary technicians to fully utilize their microscopes and increase the efficiency of viewing hematology, urinalysis, and cytology slides.

A working understanding of the available clinical instrumentation and the procedures necessary to provide accurate clinical laboratory values is necessary—in fact, required—to best serve the interests of the patient. Veterinarians will make better decisions based on their physical exam, history, and diagnostic skills without any clinical pathology data than they will if they are given erroneous data. No clinical pathology data is far better than trying to interpret erroneous data. The following are the primary responsibilities of the veterinary technician placed in charge of laboratory equipment:

1. Institute and monitor a quality control system.
2. Maintain maintenance protocols.
3. Develop standard operating procedures for all tests performed in the laboratory.
4. Provide consistent training for all individuals who will be using the equipment in the laboratory.

Currently, there are several hematology instruments available for the in-clinic laboratory. It is often the responsibility of the veterinary technician to review the instruments available prior to the investment of a large amount of money. An understanding of the types of instruments available and the differences in methods used by each instrument in obtaining data will greatly increase the potential for making an appropriate choice.

Hematology Instruments

There are basically three types of instruments available for the veterinary clinic: centrifugal, impedance, and laser-based. The centrifugal system uses a large-bore capillary tube with a special float that expands the buffy coat when the tube is spun. The tube is coated with an eosin stain that will stain DNA and RNA. The differential uptake of the stain by white blood cells and erythrocytes allows the instrument to separate the populations in the expanded buffy coat. In the erythrocyte population, immature erythrocytes (**reticulocytes**) will take up the stain for RNA and, therefore, an estimate of reticulocyte number is possible. Once the sample is spun, white blood cell and platelet counts are estimated based on the height of each portion of the buffy coat that corresponds to each cell type and the average size of the cell type. The packed cell volume (PCV) is determined by measuring the height of the red cell column as a percentage of the total blood column in the tube.

Studies evaluating the accuracy of this methodology have shown good correlation with standard impedance instruments when samples from healthy animals are analyzed. When samples from ill animals are compared, the expanded buffy coat has poor correlation with other methods and with blood film analysis. Many pathological changes in blood interfere with an accurate evaluation of blood parameters using this methodology because alterations in cells result in abnormal layering during centrifugation.

The impedance cell counters use the principle that cells are poor conductors of an electric current. In an impedance counter, individual cells are counted as they flow through an electric field. In addition, the size of cells can be measured because the magnitude of the change in current is proportional to the cell size. This methodology has been the mainstay of automated hematology for over 50 years. It is precise and accurate in counting leukocytes, erythrocytes, and platelets and can produce a reliable but limited automated differential.

Laser-based flow cytometry instruments depend on a cell's ability to scatter light as it passes through a sheath of diluent. The degree and direction of light scatter from the laser indicates the size and "complexity" of the cell. Based on these attributes, the laser-based instrument can provide up to a 5-part automated differential. The inherent variability in light stability of individual lasers can affect the precision of the instrument.

Regardless of the methodology, blood film review is an essential part of the use of hematology instrumentation. It is an excellent internal control. When comparing what is seen on the blood film to what the instrument measures, well-trained veterinary technicians can and should trust their eyes over the instrument.

Clinical Chemistry Equipment

The currently available in-clinic chemistry instruments are primarily closed systems that utilize either "wet" or "dry" chemistry methods. The wet chemistry systems are based on traditional spectrophotometric methods with individual tests or test profiles contained in a cartridge with separate cells containing all the reagents needed for the individual test reaction. The serum (or, in some cases, plasma) is introduced into the cartridge and parsed to each cell. There is little possibility for user error other than storage of reagents, sample handling, and instrument maintenance. There are in-clinic wet chemistry units that are smaller versions of the large clinical chemistry instruments that require reconstitution of individual reagents for each test. In these instruments, the reagents and serum/plasma sample are pipetted into a reaction cell. These instruments require significant training to maintain adequate performance because there is more possibility for user (technician) error in managing the reagents, instrument, and sampling.

Dry chemistry instruments use the principle of reflected light rather than transmitted light (as used for spectrophotometric methods). This method is less affected by both hemolysis and lipemia than spectrophotometric methods. Dry chemistry instruments use slides or reagent "sticks" that contain a pad of dried reagent onto which

the serum/plasma sample is placed. Once the appropriate reaction time has passed, the amount of a specific type of reflected light is measured.

Considerations in Purchasing an Instrument

In most cases, the purchase of a clinical hematology or chemistry instrument is a major decision. There are several aspects to consider as this decision is made. One of the most important questions is how many samples will be run on the instrument each day. In most cases, greater than 5 CBC or clinical chemistry panels a day are necessary to warrant in-house instrumentation. The more often the instrument is used the more familiar the staff will be with the procedures needed to provide accurate data. Other considerations include the following:

1. Cost analysis for tests performed
   a. Cost of reagents (include 10% additional reagent costs for rerunning samples if needed)
   b. Cost of consumables (pipette tips, cuvettes)
   c. Cost of technician time
   d. Cost of overhead (electricity, building expenses)
   e. Cost of quality control product
2. Available workspace for the instrument
3. Technical skill of the individuals performing the tests
4. Sample size required (the smaller the better for many small animals)
5. Test performance time
6. Monitoring requirements for the instrument
   a. Quality control needs
   b. Maintenance time and cost
7. Technical support and cost of service contracts

Evaluation of Instrumentation

Prior to purchase, the clinical staff should be allowed to evaluate the precision and accuracy of an instrument. This is done by performing a series of evaluations, usually by serial testing of a control product or products. In most cases, 20 consecutive samplings of the control product are run and their **standard deviation** and **coefficient of variance** is determined.

To calculate a standard deviation and coefficient of variance:

1. Run a selected control product on the new instrument. Add all 20 sample values of the variable together and divide by 20. This gives you the average or mean of the data set.
2. Calculate the deviance of the data from the mean. This is done by subtracting the total mean from each individual number.
3. Square each of the individual deviations and add these squared differences.
4. Divide that sum by 19.
5. Calculate the square root of the result of the previous step. The result of this calculation is the standard deviation.
6. Calculate the **coefficient of variation** (**CV**) by dividing the standard deviation by the mean. It can be expressed either as a fraction or a percent.

For Example: In Chart 1.1, your hospital team measures the following 20 control samples and notes the following values with a mean of 2.95.

Step 1 Calculate the average of these numbers or the mean.
   a. Sum of all these numbers is 59
   b. Average of these numbers is $59/20 = 2.95$
Step 2 Calculate the deviance from each value by subtracting 2.95 from each value (see above).

Step 3 Square each of the individual deviations and add these squared differences. The sum of the squared differences is 5.21
Step 4 Divide the number you got from adding the squared differences together by 19. In this case:

$$5.21/19 = 0.274211$$

Step 5 Calculate the square root of the result of the previous step. The result of this calculation is the standard deviation. In this case:

$$0.274211^2 = 0.075191$$

Step 6 Calculate the coefficient of variance by dividing the standard deviation by the mean. In this case:

$$0.075191/2.95 = 0.0255 \text{ or } 2.55\%$$

A low coefficient of variance indicates good instrument precision ($<5\%$). In addition, running 20 samples of the control product over a period of 10 to 20 days will measure the long-term stability of the instrument. Once the 20 samples are obtained over 20 days, the coefficient of variance should be evaluated again. This will allow the hospital team to determine whether the coefficient varies over time, affecting overall precision.

Once precision is determined, the results of a specific set of tests on 20 patients can be compared to a reference laboratory to determine the instrument's correlation to standard methods. It is very important to make sure that the reference laboratory to which the comparison samples are sent uses the same methodology as the in-clinic instrument. If the methods differ, the values may not be similar, especially the liver and pancreatic enzyme values. Together these two evaluation methods will help determine the accuracy of the instrument's readings. The importance of determining both

Chart 1.1

Sample #	Value	Step 2 Calculate the deviance from the data (sample value: 2.95).	Step 3 Square each of the differences.
1	3.2	0.25	0.0625
2	3.0	0.05	0.0025
3	2.8	−0.15	0.0225
4	2.4	−0.55	0.3025
5	2.6	−0.35	0.1225
6	2.4	−0.55	0.3025
7	2.9	−0.05	0.0025
8	3.6	0.65	0.4225
9	3.8	0.85	0.7225
10	2.5	−0.45	0.2025
11	3.1	0.15	0.0225
12	3.0	0.05	0.0025
13	3.7	0.75	0.5625
14	2.5	−0.45	0.2025
15	2.2	−0.75	0.5625
16	4.2	1.25	1.5625
17	2.8	−0.15	0.0225
18	2.7	−0.25	0.0625
19	2.8	−0.15	0.0225
20	2.8	−0.15	0.0225
Sum	59		5.1

precision and correlation is illustrated in Figure 1.3.

An instrument's precision can be evaluated as one of three types: precise but not correlated with a target method, imprecise but correlated with the target method, or both precise and well correlated to the target method (the optimal scenario). When purchasing an instrument, the instrument company's technical staff should assist in performing these important evaluations. It is in their best interest to prove the utility of their instruments in providing accurate and reliable data.

Quality Control—Minimizing Analytic Error

Once an instrument has demonstrated good precision and correlation, it is the ongoing responsibility of the veterinary technician

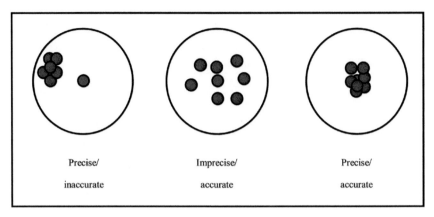

Figure 1.3.   Target illustrations of test values (red) and target value (gray) relationships. Shown are an instrument with good precision but poor correlation with the target test value, an instrument that shows correlation but poor precision, and an instrument that is both precise and has good correlation with the target value.

who supervises the laboratory to insure the continuance of accurate data. This is done by close monitoring of a well-defined in-house quality control system. All reference laboratories must employ a quality control system to monitor the overall performance of the instruments in the laboratory. A quality control system is much more than simply running a control product through an instrument at a standard interval to check the performance of the individual instrument. Quality control systems include the following:

1. A set of standard operating procedures (SOPs) for all tests performed by the veterinary technician, for evaluation of daily quality control data and actions to determine the cause of failed control data, and for appropriate training of all personnel that use the instruments
2. Maintenance records for all instruments
3. Documentation of all samples run, including name of operator, date, patient identity, results, lot number of controls, and calibrators
4. Quality control log to track daily quality control values and all actions taken

when the controls are not within the established control ranges
5. Guidelines for maintenance of the laboratory environment

Standard Operating Procedures

Standard operating procedures are often neglected in clinical practices. An SOP can be an active document if written well. The document should be written with the goal of providing anyone with the basic background in clinical pathology all the information needed to perform a specific test. The SOP is usually written in an outline form to include the following:

- Title (specific procedure)
- Scope (what is the goal of the procedure)
- Definitions pertinent to understanding the procedure
- Training level required of person performing the test
- Necessary equipment and reagents (and location)
- Procedure (step-by-step instructions)

- Quality control procedures specific to the test
- Any logs associated with procedure or instruments used in the procedure

Instrument procedure manuals can be used to supplement procedures performed by each instrument rather than duplicating the information.

Daily Quality Control

All clinical pathology results can be affected by three types of errors: preanalytical (sample handling), analytical (instrument errors), and postanalytical (reporting errors, interpretive errors). Sample handling and results reporting will be discussed later in this chapter.

All hematology instrumentation requires daily quality control measurements. The need for daily clinical chemistry quality control measurements vary between instruments. Some dry chemistry instrument manufacturers suggest that their instruments need only weekly, rather than daily, QC checks. However, if the instrument is in control limits on a given day but out of control limits 1 week later, there is no way to determine when the instrument shifted. Therefore, daily quality control is the best insurance that the clinical instruments are performing in a consistent manner.

The quality control product used should be similar to the sample being tested. For hematology systems, commercial quality control products consisting of stabilized whole blood are used. For chemistry instruments, the control product is usually a lyophilized serum–based product. In both cases, extensive analysis of each lot of control product is performed by the manufacturer to provide expected ranges for each parameter with stability over a set time once the product is opened for use. It is important to remember that control products are different than calibrators.

Calibrators are products used to set the electronics of the instrument and "tell" it what signal corresponds to a given value. In-clinic instruments are usually calibrated by the manufacturer with periodic calibrations as needed if the instrument fails to perform correctly. Control products are sample equivalents with the same physical properties as the patient's sample. The manufacturer of the clinical instrument should be able to assist in identifying appropriate commercial quality control products for use in their instrument. There are references in the literature that discuss the use of "pooled" serum samples that have been analyzed in the clinic as "control" products. Although this is a much less expensive method compared to buying commercial control products, the stability and validity of this type of quality control is questionable. **The commitment of the practice to providing quality clinical pathology data should include the use of good commercial control products with well-documented reference values and stability.**

Large reference laboratories use quality control "rules" such as the Westgard rules that employ multiple control values for each run, depending on the number of samples being run at any one time. In-house laboratories rely on quality control usually run at the beginning of each day to determine whether the instruments are working appropriately. Optimally, two to three control products are measured, one with values within the reference range for each parameter and the others with values above or below the reference range. The use of multiple control levels allows better use of rules in evaluation of quality control values. A simplified set of Westgard rules can be used when multiple control levels are evaluated with each run. When evaluating control values, it is not enough to just look at the individual value. Each new control value should be inspected in reference to the previous values. The following set of rules will assist in determining whether the instrument measurement is not stable:

1. One control value is outside 2 SD (warning rule). Repeat control measurement. If the second control value is within control reference range and none of the following rules apply, the instrument is stable. Instrument measurement is not stable if one value is outside 2 SD (warning rule) and one of the following also applies.
2. Two consecutive values are outside 2 SD on the same side of the mean.
3. The range between two consecutive values is greater than 4 SD.
4. Four consecutive values exceed 1 SD on the same side of the mean.
5. Ten consecutive values are above or below the mean.

If, using the above rules, the instrument measurement is determined to be unstable, measures should be taken to determine the cause. In most cases, the steps involved in determining the cause of erroneous control data include the following:

1. Running a new set of controls from the same lot as the original control.
2. Running a new set of controls from a new lot.
3. Performing any maintenance procedures as needed and rerunning controls after the maintenance is performed. Most instruments have a troubleshooting guide that will assist in determining the cause of instrument error.
4. Contacting the instrument's technical service if the procedures above do not reestablish the appropriate performance of the instrument.

No patient sample can be run on the instrument until it is performing appropriately and providing control data values within the expected range.

Documenting quality control can be done by daily recording the results of each quality control test performed in a quality control log. Alternatively, a graphic representation of the control data can be used. This is usually done with a Levy-Jennings graph. Figure 1.4 illustrates the use of this type of graph to recognize two distinct changes

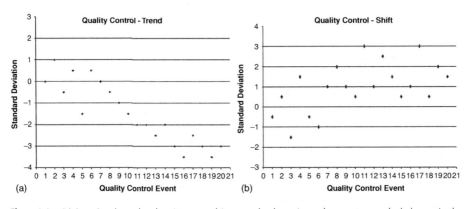

Figure 1.4. **(a)** Levy-Jennings plot showing a trend in control values. A trend suggests a gradual change in the instruments reading for a parameter in a control product. A common cause of this change is deterioration of the control product. Opening a new control product in the same lot or using a new lot may be needed to bring the values back toward the mean. **(b)** Levy-Jennings plot showing a shift in control values. A shift suggests an abrupt change in the instruments reading for a parameter in a control product. A common cause of this change is loss of calibration for that parameter. Recalibrating the instrument would be warranted.

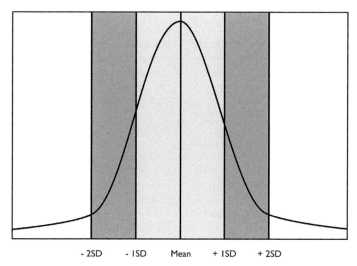

- 2SD   - ISD   Mean   + ISD   + 2SD

Figure 1.5. A distribution curve from a normal population. Shown are the mean (heavy black line) and limits for 1, 2, and 3 standard deviations from the mean of the population. Reference values for a control product are generated from this type of distribution curve by measuring the control product many times and determining the values representing the limits that include all values falling between two standard deviations from the mean. For example: If the mean for hemoglobin concentration for a control product 12.3 and the mean ±2 std is 12.9 and 11.7, respectively, then the expected value for hemoglobin in that control product should be between 11.7 to 12.9 gm/dL.

in control data, shifts, and trends. The advantage of the Levy-Jennings graph is the ability to visualize change over time that can warn the technician that intervention may be needed soon. As such, the technician will be able to take actions to keep the instruments on track before the controls indicate failure. Levy-Jennings graphs can be made using standard graph paper and the expected results and standard deviations provided with the control products used. A chart for each analyte or parameter is needed.

The expected range for a control product is determined by the manufacturer by repeated measurement of the control with calculation of the mean and standard deviation. The reference range is usually the mean value plus or minus two standard deviations (Figure 1.5). Setting the range to include all values within these limits will include 95% of the results obtained from that

control product. This means that 5% of the time, when measuring this control product, the results will be either above or below the expected range. As a result, measurements outside the range should be expected periodically.

Reference Ranges

Large laboratories usually develop their own reference ranges for each specific test using a large number of samples from healthy animals of each species for which they offer tests. This is a costly, time-consuming procedure that is essential for appropriate interpretation of laboratory data. For most small in-clinic laboratories, this process is not realistic. In most cases, the instruments in the clinic laboratory use standardized reagents and come with well-established reference ranges for all analytes tested.

However, it is still appropriate for the clinician and/or technician to review the veterinary literature for published studies that support the instrument manufacturer's claim of validation for its methods using veterinary samples. This independent validation for an instrument may point out individual parameters that are not as reliable as others measured by the instrument. For example, most in-clinic hematology instruments provide reliable erythrocyte measurements but vary significantly in the reliability of their leukocyte differential, especially when counting monocytes and eosinophils. A clinic can use wellness exams and presurgical blood work from patients undergoing elective surgeries, such as spays and neuters, to collect data over time to compare to the reference ranges provided by the instrument manufacturer. Forty to sixty samples per species can be used to generate reference ranges for the population of patients seen at a specific clinic.

Sample Handling—Minimizing Preanalytic Error

The first step in collecting any sample for clinical evaluation is adequate labeling of all containers and slides with the patient's name and the date. This is an extremely important step in sample handling that is often neglected in veterinary medicine. Close attention to sample labeling will ensure that the correct results are reported for each patient. Many clinic management software programs include label-making programs for the in-house pharmacy that can easily be used for clinical samples. The use of glass slides with a frosted end will allow labeling with a pencil. Placing labels on glass slides prior to staining can result in loss of the information during the staining procedure.

The adage "garbage in, garbage out" is very appropriate in the clinical pathology laboratory. Samples for evaluation will provide useful information only when obtained and processed correctly. Blood samples should be collected using the needle with the largest bore available to minimize the possibility of hemolysis, especially in ill animals that may have fragile erythrocytes.

The age-old controversy over the use of syringes versus vacutainer systems is not expected to end any time soon. The best compromise is to try both and use the method that is most comfortable for each individual and provides the best sample. Figure 1.6 illustrates venipuncture using a syringe.

Butterfly catheters with a connector for vacutainer tubes have nicely addressed the problem of vein collapse because of excess vacuum in patients with compromised blood pressure (Figure 1.7) and of trauma to the vein if the animal struggles. The primary advantage to using the vacutainer system is the standard volume that is drawn into the collection tube. This is extremely important when drawing blood for coagulation studies that require a precise ratio of coagulant to blood.

Whole blood for a complete blood count (CBC) must be collected in an anticoagulant. EDTA is the most common anticoagulant used for this purpose. It is essential that the blood be promptly mixed to prevent the formation of clots that will interfere with cell counting. Heparin can be used in certain cases, but it interferes with staining of the blood cells for blood film analysis. The ratio of blood to anticoagulant is important, as mentioned above. If too little blood is drawn into the collection tube, the anticoagulant, if in liquid form, will cause dilution of the blood resulting in artifactual low values.

In addition, erythrocytes will shrink due to the high osmolality (solute concentration) of the anticoagulant fluid. This can result in artifactual changes in red cell shape when the blood film is reviewed, in an

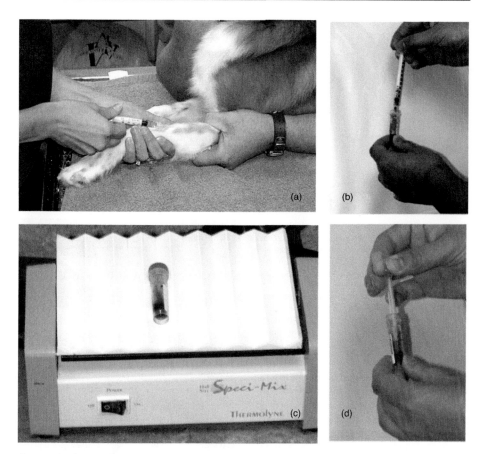

Figure 1.6. The steps for venipuncture using a syringe method. **(a)** The patient's forearm is held off and the technical team member draws blood from the cephalic artery. The needle should be at least 22 gauge or larger to prevent hemolysis. **(b)** Once the blood is drawn, it is placed into the EDTA blood tube; care should be taken to remove the top of the tube and expel the blood directly into the tube. This helps to reduce hemolysis. The EDTA tube should be inverted 7–8 times so that the blood and EDTA can properly mix. **(c)** If possible, place the sample on a sample rocker to allow the blood samples to continue to mix properly with the EDTA. **(d)** Finally, before making the blood smear, a small section of the sample should be examined with a pipette or wooden applicator sticks to make sure there is no obvious clot formation. If clotting is observed, this sample should be disposed of and a new sample obtained.

artifactual decrease in the packed cell volume (PCV), and in discordance between the PCV and the hematocrit (Hct) value in the automated CBC. In this case, the instrument Hct will be the more accurate value because the erythrocytes will "rehydrate" when the instrument performs the necessary dilution of the blood sample for counting.

If too much blood is placed into the collection tube, clots will form. The clots in this case may be too small to visualize but can affect the results and may cause

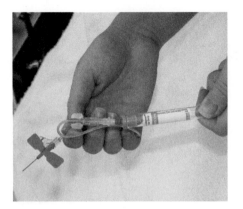

Figure 1.7. The use of a butterfly catheter with a vacutainer adapter often makes the collection of blood easier than using a needle and syringe. After the catheter is placed it can be secured to the patient, diminishing the chances of damaging the vessel if the patient struggles. An additional advantage is that this method allows the collection of a small amount of blood for a quick PCV, total protein, and blood film while clearing the catheter and tubing of blood that may contain procoagulant factors that would promote clot formation in the EDTA tube.

obstruction of the tubing within the instrument causing instrument failure. Gross inspection of the blood for clots is essential prior to introducing a sample into an instrument. In addition to checking for clots, the presence of agglutination should be noted if present. Agglutination will artifactually alter most erythrocyte indices reported by the instrument. Since a total protein and a PCV are important aspects of a complete blood count and should be performed on all whole blood samples, the appearance of the buffy coat can be recorded as well. A thick buffy coat supports the presence of a **leukocytosis** or **thrombocytosis**; a thin buffy coat indicates a **leukopenia** or **thrombocytopenia**; and reddish discoloration suggests possible **reticulocytosis**. Young erythrocytes are less dense than mature erythrocytes and can sediment out in the buffy coat when the blood is spun.

Making a good blood film is essential to blood film analysis. There are several techniques used to make good blood films. There is no absolute correct method. Two methods are illustrated in Figure 1.8. The best method to use is the one that allows the individual to produce the best blood film. Try as many methods as possible, and review the blood films for even distribution of **leukocytes** and the presence of an adequate counting area. Adopt the one that works best for each individual. The only method that is discouraged is the used of the "pull" preparation normally used for cytology preparation (see Chapter 15).

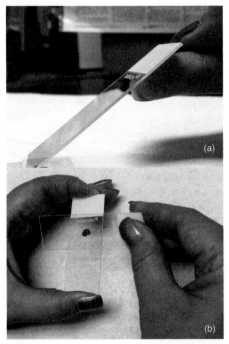

(a)

(b)

Figure 1.8. Two methods for preparing a blood film. **(a)** The push slide is rested on one finger rather than being held between the thumb and index finger. The method prevents excessive pressure on the push slide. Excessive pressure results in uneven distribution of the leukocytes to the feathered edge. **(b)** Both the push slide and blood film slide are in the hands. This technique allows some individuals better control of the slides. There are additional techniques for blood film preparation. Try as many methods as possible and choose the one that produces the best blood film.

The methods of blood film evaluation and estimates for leukocyte and platelet numbers were developed for the distribution of these cells in the traditionally prepared blood film. One important note on preparing blood films is to note that the angle of the "push" slide needed to provide a good blood film depends on the viscosity of the blood. Thin (anemic patient) blood requires a steep angle or the blood film may run off the end of the slide. Thick blood (dehydrated patient) requires a shallow angle or the blood film will be too short and there will be an inadequate counting area (Figure 1.9).

Practice is the only way to develop good blood film—making skills. Figure 1.10 illustrates common problems in blood film preparation.

The most common stain used in practice is a modified quick **Romanowsky stain (Diff-Quik)**. Romanowsky-type stains differentially stain the cytoplasm of the leukocytes. The azure or blue dye stains the acid components of the cells (nuclei and proteins), the eosin or red dye stains the basic components of the cell (carbohydrates, some granules). The pH of the stains is critical. Therefore, keeping the stains fresh and limiting evaporation are important in maintaining the pH of the solutions.

Stains should be changed frequently (at least every 2 weeks if used often). There are a number of Romanowsky-type stains available to the practice. The most commonly used stain in reference laboratories is the Wright-Giemsa or Modified Wright-Giemsa stain. These have the advantage of providing a truer staining quality to reticulocytes on a blood film and are preferred for staining cytological preparation of lymph nodes and other lymphoid organs. Spending the time to evaluate different stains is recommended.

Samples collected for clinical chemistry tests are usually collected in collection tubes without anticoagulant and allowed to clot for at least 15–20 minutes. Following clot-

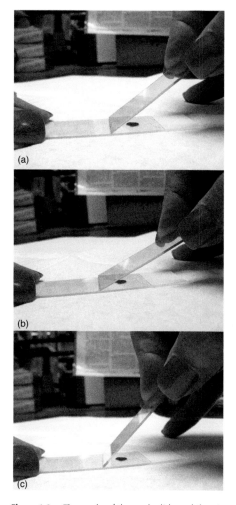

Figure 1.9. The angle of the push slide and the viscosity of the blood determine the length of the blood film. **(a)** For blood with a normal PCV, a 45° angle will produce a blood film with a good feathered edge and counting area. **(b)** For blood that is thick (dehydration), a shallower angle is needed or the blood film will be too short. **(c)** For blood that is thin (anemia), a steeper angle is needed or the blood film will be too long.

ting the sample is centrifuged and the serum is pipetted off, or, if a serum separator tube is used, poured off and placed in a clean tube and sealed tightly. Occasionally,

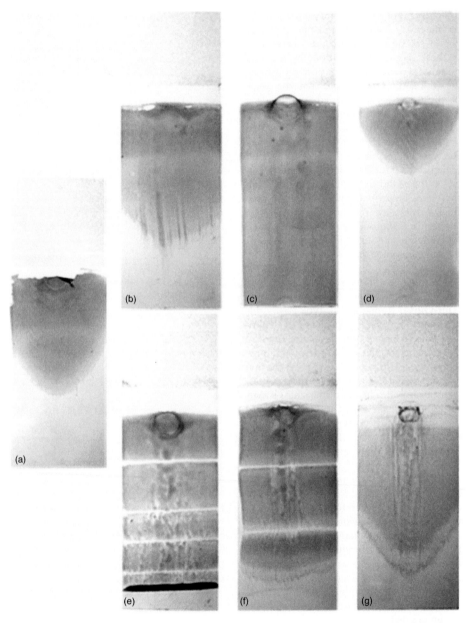

Figure 1.10. Blood film examples. **(a)** An example of a well-made blood film. **(b)** Streaks in the blood film due to platelet clumps or dust on the slide. **(c)** Too much blood dropped on the slide or the angle of the push slide is too low. **(d)** Too little blood dropped on the slide or the angle of the push slide is too high. **(e)** Hesitation with abrupt lifting of the push slide at the end. **(f)** Hesitation. **(g)** Drops of blood allowed to sit too long before making the slide.

samples are collected in heparin and plasma is collected. This is usually done when the volume of the blood sample is expected to be small, such as with puppies, kittens, or pocket pets and in severely dehydrated patients. The volume of plasma obtained from a blood sample is often greater than for serum.

In addition, the sample can be centrifuged immediately for testing rather than waiting for clot formation. It is important to remember that not all chemistry tests can be performed on heparinized plasma and that the correct type of heparin must be used (lithium heparin). It is essential that the serum or plasma portion of the blood is separated from the cellular portion as soon as possible. Delayed separation of the blood sample can cause significant artifactual changes in several chemistry parameters. The tests most consistently affected by prolonged exposure of the serum or plasma to cells are glucose and phosphorus. Potassium concentration can also be significantly increased over time in patients with increased platelet numbers and in certain breeds such as the Akita due to active transport of potassium out the cells into the serum.

As with whole blood samples for hematology, serum samples should be examined and changes in color and clarity recorded. The presence of **lipemia, hemolysis,** and **icterus** should be noted in the record when present. Most clinical chemistry instruments will provide information concerning what individual clinical chemistry tests are affected by lipemia, hemolysis, and icterus. It is important to note these effects when reporting results for a sample with these changes.

For urine samples, the method of collection should always be recorded. Interpretation of the result of the urinalysis will be greatly affected by the method used. Optimally, cystocentesis and catheterization are the preferred methods of urine collection. Collection and storage of the urine sample in a clean, sterile container will allow culture of the sample if the urinalysis results suggest a possible septic process. Urine samples can be stored in the refrigerated for 24 hours if the sample cannot be processed within 1–4 hours. If the sample is refrigerated, it must be allowed to reach room temperature prior to analysis. The artifactual effects of urine sample handling will be further outlined in Chapter 9.

The veterinary technician plays a pivotal role in the provision of clinical laboratory data in the veterinary practice. To do this, an understanding of how laboratory data is produced (instrumentation), an understanding of the basic physiology behind disease processes, and experience and training in blood film evaluation will allow the technician to provide excellent data, recognize incongruent laboratory values, and anticipate further testing by the veterinarian.

Although the veterinarian is the individual responsible for interpretation of data during the process of diagnosis and treatment follow-up, the technician is the individual that is responsible for overseeing the provision of accurate data and troubleshooting the process when problems arise. The following chapters focus on providing an overview of hematology, clinical chemistry, urinalysis, and cytology that will enable the veterinary technician to be a proactive part in practical clinical pathology.

Components of the Complete Blood Count

The **complete blood count (CBC)** is a process by which the cellular components of the blood are evaluated. The components of the CBC provide data that is used to determine whether there are abnormalities in **erythrocytes**, leukocytes, and platelets. The packed cell volume (PCV), hematocrit (Hct), hemoglobin concentration, and indices that describe the size of erythrocytes and the concentration of hemoglobin within the erythrocytes are used to evaluate erythrocytes.

The white blood cell count (WBC) and differential leukocyte count are used to evaluate leukocytes. The blood film evaluation is an essential part of the CBC and is used to confirm the numbers obtained by the automated or manual CBC and to fully evaluate cell morphology. The CBC can be automated or performed manually. The automated CBC includes each of the above components, while the majority of manual CBCs do not include measurement of hemoglobin or the erythrocyte indices.

The necessary items for a manual CBC are shown in Figure 2.1. Because it can be difficult to fully interpret the results of a CBC without a total protein, this measurement should be included as an important component of the CBC. The total protein can be measured by refractometer or by an in-house chemistry instrument.

The Hemogram

The **hemogram** is the collection of specific measurements that allow the veterinarian to evaluate a patient's erythrocytes, leukocytes, and platelets. The portion of the hemogram that contains the parameters that assess erythrocytes is the erythrogram and the portion that relates to the leukocytes is the leukogram. Platelet parameters are often reported with the erythrogram. Most automated cell counters will provide the following measurements:

- Red cell count measured in cells/μL
- **Hematocrit (Hct)** measured in percent
- **Mean cell volume (MCV)** measured in femtoliters (fl)

19

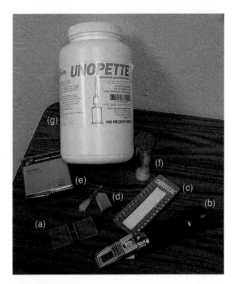

Figure 2.1. **(a)** Hemocytometer. **(b)** Refractometer. **(c)** Microhematocrit tube sealant. **(d)** Unopette system diluent reservoir and pipette. **(e)** Microscope slides. **(f)** Microhematocrit tubes. **(g)** Unopette WBC counting system.

- **Hemoglobin (Hgb)** measured in g/dL
- **Mean cell hemoglobin concentration (MCHC)** measured in g/dL
- **Mean cell hemoglobin (MCH)** measured in pg
- Platelets numbers in cells/µL
- White blood cell count in cells/µL
- **Leukocyte differential** cell counts in percents and absolute numbers in cells/µL (Table 2.1).

The Erythrogram

The three erythrocyte parameters in the erythrogram that are directly measured by most in-clinic hematology instruments are hemoglobin, red cell count, and red cell volume. The remaining red cell parameters—MCHC, Hct, and MCH—are calculated from the measured values. As a result, if there are artifactual changes in the

measured values, the calculated values will be erroneous.

Each of these measurements can help identify and characterize the anemic patient. The definition of **anemia** is decreased circulating erythrocytes. Therefore, an anemic patient will have decreased erythrocyte count, decreased Hct, and decreased Hgb. There are occasions in which all three of these measurements are not decreased. When this happens, an investigation into why this discordance is present should be done. To understand how discordant values occur, the technician must understand how these measurements are made.

The majority of in-house hematology instruments measure hemoglobin using a spectrophotometric method. When this method is used, a fixed amount of blood is diluted in a lysing solution to release the hemoglobin from the erythrocytes. Then, a light of a specific wavelength (540 nanometers) is passed through the fluid containing the released hemoglobin, and the amount that is transmitted to the photocell on the other side of the fluid is measured (Figure 2.2).

The amount of hemoglobin present is inversely proportional to the amount of light that is transmitted. The less light that passes through the fluid, the more hemoglobin will be measured in the fluid. Therefore, anything that will decrease the amount of light that can pass through the fluid or scatters light as it passes through the fluid will cause an artifactual increase in the hemoglobin measurement. Artifactual changes in the measurement of hemoglobin will directly affect the calculation of MCHC and MCH.

The red cell count is a direct count of individual cells as they pass through an electrical field (impedance) or a flow cell (laser counters) (Figure 2.3). Erroneous red cell counts will affect the Hct and MCH. The MCV is a direct measurement of cell size that is related to the magnitude of the disrupted electrical current as each cell passes through the instrument. Erroneous

Table 2.1. Components of the hemogram.

Measurement	Component Measured	Units
Hematocrit/PCV	Measures the RBC mass as a percentage of blood. The hematocrit is calculated by an instrument and the PCV is measured.	Percent
Hemoglobin concentration	Measures the amount of hemoglobin contained in the blood	Grams/deciliter (g/dL)
Red cell count	Measures the number of red blood cells/unit volume	Million/microliter (10^6/uL)
Mean cell volume (MCV)	Measures the average volume of the individual red blood cells	Femtoliter (fl) or cubic micrometer (um^3)
Mean cell hemoglobin concentration (MCHC)	Measures the average hemoglobin concentration in individual red blood cells	Percent
Mean cell hemoglobin (MCH)	Measures the average amount of hemoglobin in the individual red blood cell	Picogram (pg)
Total white blood cell count	Measures the number of white blood cells/unit volume	Thousands/microliter (10^3/uL)
Platelet count	Measures the number of platelets/unit volume	Thousands/microliter (10^3/uL)
Neutrophil count	Measures the absolute number of neutrophils/unit volume	Thousands/microliter (10^3/uL)
Eosinophil count	Measures the absolute number of eosinophils/unit volume	Thousands/microliter (10^3/uL)
Monocyte count	Measures the absolute number of monocytes/unit volume	Thousands/microliter (10^3/uL)
Lymphocyte count	Measures the absolute number of lymphocytes/unit volume	Thousands/microliter (10^3/uL)
Basophil count	Measures the absolute number of basophils/unit volume	Thousands/microliter (10^3/uL)
% neutrophils	The percentage of neutrophils in the total white count	Percent
% eosinophils	The percentage of eosinophils in the total white count	Percent
% monocytes	The percentage of monocytes in the total white count	Percent
% lymphocytes	The percentage of lymphocytes in the total white count	Percent
% basophils	The percentage of basophils in the total white count	Percent

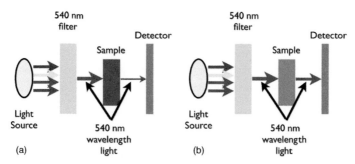

Figure 2.2.   The components of a simple spectrophotometer. The filter allows one wavelength from the light source to pass through, 540 nm in the case of hemoglobin measurement. The hemoglobin in the sample will absorb the light in proportion to the amount of hemoglobin. The more hemoglobin in the sample, the less light will pass through to the detector. Anything that will interfere with light passing through a solution will erroneously increase the instruments measurement of hemoglobin. **(a)** The sample has a high concentration of hemoglobin, absorbs a large amount of the 540 nm wavelength and, therefore, a small amount of the light passes through the sample for detection. **(b)** This sample has a low concentration of hemoglobin and, therefore, a large amount of the light passes through the sample for detection.

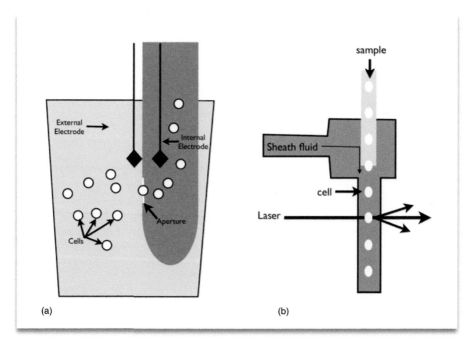

Figure 2.3.   Schematic of an impedance counter (a) and a laser counter (b). **(a)** In the impedance counter, an electrical current is created across a small opening (the aperture) by the external and internal electrodes. As the cells are aspirated through the aperture, they disrupt the current in proportion to the size of the cell. As a result, both the number and size of the cells are measured. **(b)** In the laser counter, cells flow through a channel in single file and pass through a single beam of focused light. The light is scattered to a different degree by the different types of cells.

measurement of the MCV will affect the Hct and MCHC.

The platelet count is usually reported with the erythrogram. Platelets are directly counted in most instruments. They are counted in the same cycle as the erythrocytes. The two populations are separated by their size. In those instruments that use impedance, a histogram (a distribution curve) shows the size difference between the platelets and erythrocytes. The instrument must be able to identify a valley between the two populations to produce an accurate platelet count.

In some cases, large platelets (**macroplatelets**) may interfere with the count. Large platelets are produced when platelets are being consumed. Cavalier King Charles spaniels can have large platelets as a breed characteristic. Figure 2.4 shows three histograms, one from a patient with normal-sized platelets, one from a patient with small erythrocytes, and one from a patient with macroplatelets. Platelet clumps will

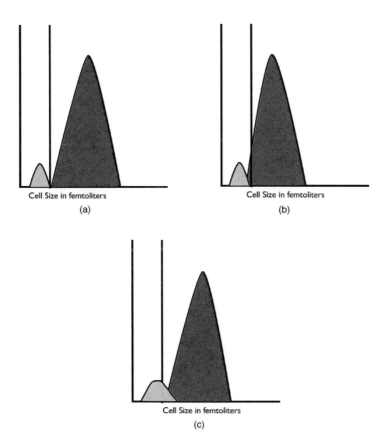

Figure 2.4. Red blood cell and platelet histograms. **(a)** Normal histogram showing a well-defined "valley" between the platelets and the red blood cells. **(b)** Histogram from an individual with small red blood cells that extend into the platelet size ranges, making it difficult for the instrument to accurately count the platelets. **(c)** Histogram from an individual with large platelets. In this case, the larger platelets will be counted as red blood cells and an artifactually low platelet count will be reported.

also interfere with the platelet count. Small clusters of platelets are lost in the red cell population and, therefore, not counted as platelets. The larger clusters are not counted at all. Evaluation of the blood film is necessary for identification of macroplatelets and platelet clumps and interpretation of the platelet count.

The Leukogram

The total white blood cell count, leukocyte differential, absolute leukocyte counts, and leukocyte morphology abnormalities are all components of the leukogram. The total white blood cell count and, in some instruments, the absolute number of individual cell types are direct counts. Although there are in-clinic instruments that offer automated differential and absolute differential cell counts, blood films should be reviewed to confirm the number and distribution of leukocytes.

This can be done quickly by examining the slide at 10 for overall cellularity and at 40× to confirm the differential. If on review of the blood film, there is concern for the accuracy of the instrument differential cell count and absolute numbers, a manual differential should be done. In most cases, a 100 cell differential suffices. However, if the total cell count is greater than 30,000/µL, a 200 cell differential should be done. The more cells counted in the differential cell count, the more accurate the count. An essential part of the leukogram is the morphological evaluation of the leukocytes. Comments on the presence of toxic change and Dohlé bodies, reactive lymphocytes, and atypical or unidentified cells should be noted where appropriate. These changes will be discussed in Chapter 4.

The manual differential cell count is the most time-consuming component of the CBC. The process can be shortened considerably by the use of a differential cell counter. Two types of differential cell counters are shown in Figure 2.5.

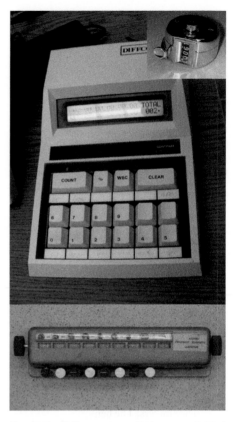

Figure 2.5. Cell counters. Bottom, mechanical counter; top, electronic counter; inset: individual cell counter.

The digital counter has the advantage of calculating the absolute numbers from the percentages obtained in the differential cell count. In addition, most digital counters have a key to count nucleated erythrocytes (nRBC) without affecting the differential. If the technician is using the mechanical counter, an additional single counter will be needed to keep track of the nRBC. The single counter is also used to count cells on the hemocytometer when performing the manual WBC.

Manual white blood cell counts may be needed in some cases, such as when the amount of blood obtained is insufficient for

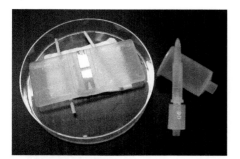

Figure 2.6. Hemocytometer and Unopette system for manually counting white blood cells.

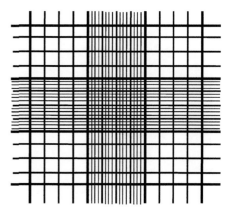

Figure 2.7. Neubauer grid for counting cells.

an automated count or the blood film does not verify the automated WBC. Manual cell counts are most commonly done using the Unopette system and a hemocytometer (Figure 2.6).

There are several types of Unopette systems available. Table 2.2 lists the systems most commonly used for white blood cell counts. If more than one system is used in the clinic, it is important to be sure that the pipettes are used only with the correct diluent reservoir. The pipettes measure a specific volume that is different for each dilution reservoir. There are several types of hemocytometers. The hemocytometers with the improved Neubauer grid are the most commonly used type (Figure 2.7). The coverslip that accompanies the hemocytometer is specifically weighted for use with the hemocytometer. Extra coverslips should

be purchased to have on hand in case of breakage.

The following is a short protocol for performing a WBC using a hemocytometer and the Unopette system:

1. Place the blood sample on the sample rocker to mix thoroughly (Figure 2.8a).
2. Clean the grid surface of the hemocytometer and the coverslip with water and a dust-free tissue (lens paper works well). Wipe both dry. Be gentle with the fragile coverslips. They are usually broken when being cleaned.
3. Place the coverslip over the counting area of the hemocytometer.
4. Using the pipette cover, pierce the diaphragm of the reservoir to open it (Figure 2.8b).
5. Charge the Unopette pipette with blood. Capillary action will draw the blood up to the hub of the pipette. Carefully wipe off the outside of the pipette being sure not to touch the tip of the pipette with the tissue (Figures 2.8c,d).
6. Squeeze the Unopette reservoir slightly and carefully seat the pipette tip firmly into the neck of the reservoir. Release the reservoir to allow the vacuum to pull the blood into the

Table 2.2. Types of Unopette systems.

Method	Contents
Leukocyte count	3% acetic acid (cannot be used to count cells in joint fluid)
Platelet/leukocyte count	1% ammonium oxalate
Reticulocyte stain set	New methylene blue

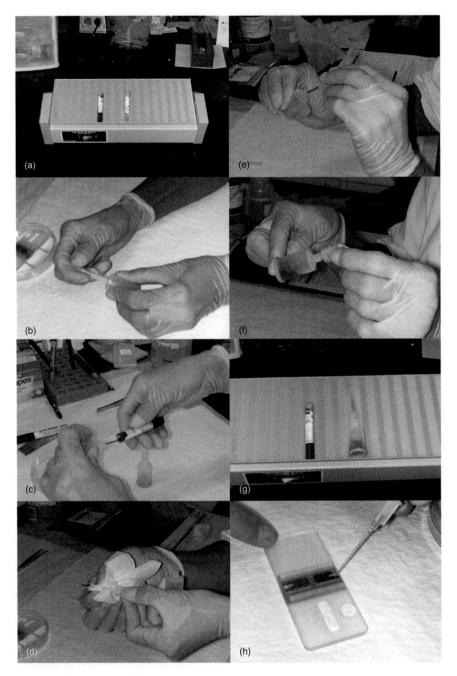

Figure 2.8. Performing a manual WBC count.

dilution fluid. Gently rinse the pipette by slightly squeezing and releasing the reservoir to force fluid into the pipette without spilling fluid from the open end of the pipette (Figures 2.8e,f).

7. Allow the charged reservoir to sit for 5 minutes on a rocker to allow complete lysis of the erythrocytes and to mix thoroughly. If a rocker is not available, be sure to mix the reservoir gently 10–15 times just before charging the hemocytometer (Figure 2.8g).

8. Remove the pipette and seat the hub back into the reservoir.

9. Just before placing the tip of the pipette into the charging channel on the hemocytometer, expel a few drops to clear any residue in the pipette that may not be well mixed.

10. Gently squeeze the reservoir to form a small drop and set it in the charging channel of the hemocytometer (Figure 2.8h).

11. Allow the fluid to be pulled, by capillary action, under the coverslip just until the chamber is filled. Practice may be needed to accurately charge a hemocytometer. If the chamber is overfilled or underfilled, the count will not be accurate.

12. Place the hemocytometer in a humidified chamber (Figure 2.9).

13. Place the hemocytometer on the microscope stage and view using the 10× objective. The stage will have to be lowered significantly to bring the counting grid on the hemocytometer into view. By focusing on the tip of the charging channel, it is easy to find the grid by moving the stage in the direction of the point of the channel.

14. Count all the cells in the 9 large squares following a pattern that starts in the upper-left square along the top row to the right, down to the middle row along to the left, and then down to the bottom row along to the right again.

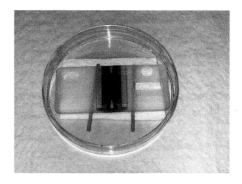

Figure 2.9. A petri dish, small absorbent paper, and two sections of an applicator stick are used to make a humidity chamber. A small amount of water is used to moisten the paper. The hemocytometer is placed in this chamber for about 5 minutes to allow the cells to settle onto the surface. Once the cover of the petri dish is in place, the moisture from the moisten paper will prevent loss of fluid from under the cover slip due to evaporation.

15. In order to keep track of the cells that fall on the lines of the grid, include the cells on the top and left lines of each square in the count for that square. Figure 2.10 illustrates the grid and how cells are counted.

16. Charge and count both sides of the hemocytometer. The counts should be within 10% of each other. Average the two counts before calculating the WBC using the formula provided by the Unopette system used.

17. Be sure to thoroughly clean the hemocytometer and coverslip before storing them.

The Blood Film

The blood film is an essential part of the complete blood count. It can be used as an internal control for the white blood cell count, differential, and platelet count. As discussed in Chapter 1, a good uniform blood film is essential to the process of blood film examination. There is an

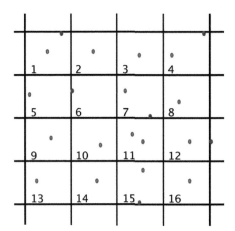

Figure 2.10. When counting the cells in the grid, it is standard practice to count the cells that are on the lines in a standard pattern to keep from counting a cell twice. The cells on the top and left of each small square are counted with that square, while the cells on the bottom and right are not. In this field, the red cell on the lines in squares 1, 4, 6, and 11 will be counted in each of their respective squares because they are on the top or left lines. The red cells on the line in squares 12 and 15 will be excluded from their respective squares because they are on the bottom line.

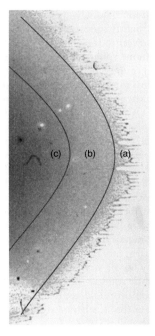

Figure 2.11. **(a)** The feathered edge. **(b)** The counting area. **(c)** The body of the film.

"anatomy" to the blood film, and each part of the blood film is used for a specific purpose.

Figure 2.11 illustrates the regions of the blood film: feathered edge, counting area, and body. As the blood film is made, large things such as platelet clumps, large atypical cells, and microfilaria are carried to the feathered edge. However, in this area, the erythrocytes and leukocytes are flattened and do not show a normal morphology. As a result, erythrocyte and leukocyte morphology cannot be evaluated in this area. Erythrocyte and leukocyte morphology evaluation is done in the counting area where the blood cells form a monolayer. In the counting area, the red cells in those species with a good central pallor, such as the dog, are easy to distinguish from atypical cells such as spherocytes, and the cytoplasm and nucleus of the leukocytes are clearly seen.

In a well-made blood film, the leukocyte distribution will allow an estimation of the WBC count and an accurate differential cell count. The body of the film is in the thicker portion of the blood film where the red cells are just overlapping. Figure 2.11 illustrates the cell density seen in each of the three areas of the blood film.

Evaluation of the blood film is done at several levels. The initial step is scanning the slide at low power (10× objective) for a quick estimate of the white blood cell count (>50 white blood cells/field indicates a high count, <20 cells/field indicates a low cell count) and review of the feathered edge for large cells, platelet clumps, and parasites (i.e., microfilaria). On low power, the quality of the blood film can be determined (i.e., is the cell distribution even or are all the cells at the feathered edge?). This quick assessment of the WBC count can be used to support the manual or automated count. A more accurate estimate of the WBC count can be done using the high dry objective (40×). When using the 40× objective, it is important to use a coverslip or the cells will not be in focus. This estimate is done in the "counting" area of the blood film. The following steps can be used for this estimate:

1. Count all leukocytes in 10 40× fields.
2. Total leukocyte counted / # of fields counted × 2000 = estimated leukocyte count
3. If the patient is anemic a corrected count can be obtained by the following formula:
   Corrected count = (estimated count × (actual PCV / normal PCV))
   (For the "normal PCV," use 45 for dogs and 35 for cats)
   Example:
   > 100 cells counted / 10 fields
   > 10 × 2000 = (approximately) 20,000/μL
   > PCV 22
   > 20,000 × (22/45) = (approximately) 9,800/μL

A similar formula can be used to estimate the platelet count. For platelets, the estimate is done using the oil immersion objective in the body of the blood film. The following steps can be used for platelet estimate:

1. Count all platelets in 10 oil immersion fields.
2. Total platelets counted / # of fields counted × 20,000 = estimated platelet count
   Example:
   > 100 platelets counted / 10 fields
   > 10 × 20,000 = (approximately) 200,000/μL
   > (Note: if the number of platelets seen in each field is 10 or greater, the patient should have a normal platelet mass).

The above estimates of the white blood cell and platelet counts are based on a standard objective working field diameter of 0.63 mm. If the working field diameter of the clinic microscope is larger or smaller, the estimates may need to be adjusted for that particular microscope.

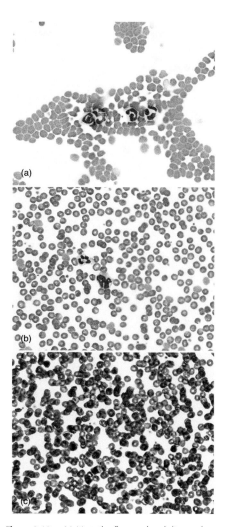

Figure 2.12. **(a)** Note the flattened and distorted erythrocytes and neutrophils at the feathered edge. **(b)** Note the central pallor in the erythrocytes and the crisp nucleus of both the neutrophil and monocyte in the counting area. **(c)** Note the increased density of the erythrocytes in the body of the blood film.

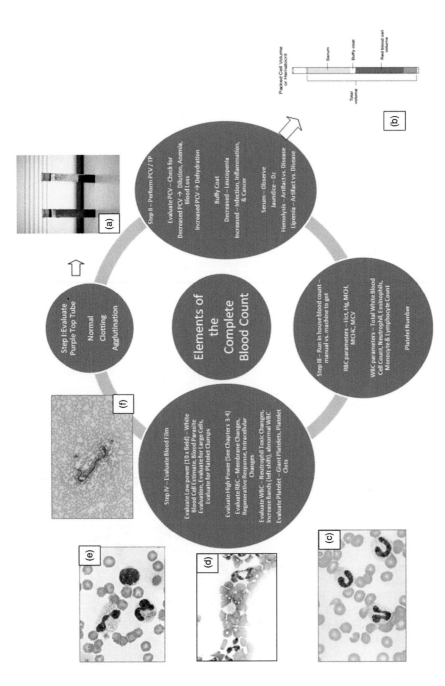

Figure 2.13. The following is an overview of the components of the CBC. Step 1 evaluates the purple top tube for abnormality; in figure **a**, the purple top tube on the right shows agglutination. Figure **b** illustrates the components of the PCV. Finally, the hospital team member must be able to evaluate the blood smear for band neutrophils (**c**), intracellular pathology (**d**), changes in cell membranes (**e**), and blood parasites (**f**) and other changes.

After the WBC and platelet counts are verified, morphological evaluation of erythrocytes, leukocytes and platelets can be done. Platelet size, changes in leukocyte morphology, and erythrocyte morphology should be noted. Leukocyte atypia and cytoplasmic abnormalities such as reactive lymphocytes and neutrophil toxicity are important findings to be noted in the CBC (Figures 2.12, 2.13). There are several changes in the erythrocyte morphology that should be reported. Changes in size (anisocytosis), shape (poikilocytosis), color (polychromasia or hypochromasia) and the presence of inclusions can be seen because of underlying disease processes. The specific abnormalities identified in the CBC will be discussed in Chapter 4.

Hematology: The Erythrocytes, White Blood Cells, and Immune System

Hematology is the study of the cellular components of blood. Blood is composed of both cells and fluid. The cells are white blood cell (leukocytes), erythrocytes (erythrocytes), and platelets. The fluid component consists of water, protein, electrolytes/minerals, lipids, soluble carbohydrates, amino acids, and other noncellular substances such as hormones. Each component of blood has a specific function and can change in response to disease states. This chapter discusses the cellular components of blood and includes normal physiology of each cell type.

Immunology is the study of the immune system. The immune system is a complex cellular defense that recognizes foreign substances and infectious agents and mounts a reaction to destroy the foreign agent. There are two primary divisions of the immune system: innate immunity and acquired immunity. The cells of the innate immune system include the peripheral blood leukocytes (neutrophils, eosinophils, and monocytes) and are discussed in the hematology section of this chapter. Acquired immunity requires

the stimulation of lymphocytes and is discussed as a separate section.

Hematology

The enumeration and morphological evaluation of the peripheral blood cells are essential parts of the complete blood count. An understanding of the formation, function, and peripheral dynamics of white blood cells will allow the veterinary technician to accurately identify and report changes in the CBC associated with disease processes.

Hematopoiesis

Hematopoiesis is the production of blood cells. All peripheral blood cells are formed in the bone marrow from a single cell, a stem cell. The stem cell produces cells that commit to a specific cell type in response to specific growth factors. Hematopoiesis

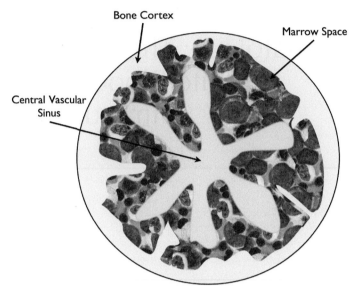

Figure 3.1. The hematopoietic tissue is present within the marrow spaces of the long bones. The mature leukocytes, erythrocytes, and platelets are released into the central sinusoids of the marrow and, eventually, into the peripheral blood. Normal supportive structures of the bone marrow are as essential to normal blood cell production as the hematopoietic cells.

is separated into **granulopoiesis** (neutrophil, eosinophil, basophil production), **erythropoiesis** (erythrocyte production), and **megakaryopoiesis** (platelet production).

Bone marrow is found within the central core of most bones throughout the body. Figure 3.1 illustrates the structure of bone marrow.

The bone marrow consists of supportive cells, their supportive matrix (the microenvironment), and hematopoietic cells. The supportive cells that provide a productive microenvironment are macrophages, fat cells, fibrocytes, and vascular endothelial cells (cells that line the blood vessels). The hematopoietic cells are uncommitted stem cells, committed stem cells, and various maturation stages of each cell type. The microenvironment is extremely important. Injury to the cells and supportive structures of the microenvironment will result in de-

creased production of blood cells. In addition to the structural support, the microenvironment must provide access to certain circulating hormones, growth factors (substances produced by supportive cells), and nutrients.

There are many factors that control hematopoiesis to maintain normal numbers of erythrocytes, white blood cells, and platelets and to increase production of each of these cell types when needed. Figure 3.2 illustrates the progression of hematopoiesis from the uncommitted (pleuripotential) stem cell that gives rise to all blood cells and primary growth factors that act to promote production of these cells.

The stimuli to increase production of each cell type are varied. For example, erythrocyte production is increased in response to hypoxia perceived by the kidney. The cells that surround the tubules of the kidney respond to changes in oxygenation

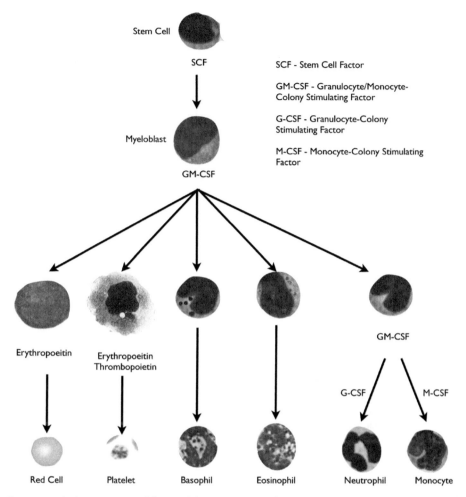

Stem Cell

SCF

Myeloblast

GM-CSF

SCF - Stem Cell Factor

GM-CSF - Granulocyte/Monocyte-Colony Stimulating Factor

G-CSF - Granulocyte-Colony Stimulating Factor

M-CSF - Monocyte-Colony Stimulating Factor

Erythropoeitin

Erythropoeitin
Thrombopoietin

GM-CSF

G-CSF   M-CSF

Red Cell   Platelet   Basophil   Eosinophil   Neutrophil   Monocyte

Figure 3.2. The hematopoietic cell lines and the primary growth factors that control production of each type of blood cell.

of the sounding tissue. **Erythropoietin,** the primary hormone that stimulates erythropoiesis, is produced at a constant rate to maintain the normal rate of erythropoiesis. The circulating concentration of erythropoietin increases when the oxygenation of the renal tissue decreases.

There are also factors that inhibit hematopoiesis. The maintenance of normal concentrations of peripheral blood cells de- pends on a balance between the factors that promote hematopoiesis and those that inhibit the process.

There are many factors that can stimulate the production of neutrophils, several of which are produced as a result of inflammation.

In the normal animal, the bone marrow produces the majority of blood cells. The spleen is another site of hematopoiesis, extramedullary hematopoiesis. The majority of blood cells produced in the spleen are erythrocytes; however, both granulocytes and platelets can also be formed in the spleen. This organ can increase its production of blood cells when needed but cannot replace the bone marrow as the primary site of hematopoiesis. Several changes in the peripheral blood occur when the spleen has increased production of erythrocytes, including increased circulating nucleated erythrocytes.

Erythropoiesis

Erythrocytes are formed in sinusoids of the bone marrow, surrounded by "nurse" cells (specialized macrophages that store iron and **phagocytize** the extruded nucleus) and move though the walls of the sinusoids into the bloodstream. Figure 3.3 illustrates the progression of the erythrocyte from the committed stem cell to the mature erythrocyte.

As the erythrocyte matures it becomes smaller, accumulates more hemoglobin, and eventually extrudes its nucleus. The number of mitotic divisions the cell undergoes is closely regulated and determines the final size of the red cell. During normal production of erythrocytes, only mature erythrocytes are released into the circulation.

With increased demand, younger, larger, polychromatophilic erythrocytes (stress reticulocytes) are released. The blue hue of the young polychromatophilic red cell is due to RNA in the cytoplasm. Once released, the reticulocyte will continue to make hemoglobin and eventually lose the RNA. **However, it does not become smaller.**

The normal life span of the erythrocyte varies between species. In the cat, normal red cells circulate for approximately 70 days; in the dog, the red cells circulate for approximately 110 days. As the red cells age, they are removed by macrophages in

the spleen and, to a lesser degree, liver and bone marrow. These cells are replaced by new red cells to maintain the normal red cell count in the peripheral blood. Erythrocyte maturation takes approximately 3–5 days. As a result, if an animal has an episode of significant blood loss, it may take up to 7 days to see any evidence of regeneration in the peripheral blood sample.

The erythrocytes only function is to carry oxygen from the lung to the tissues and CO_2 from the tissues to the lung. The shape of the cell, hemoglobin, cytoplasmic enzymes, and membrane-associated electrolyte pumps all contribute to moving oxygen from the alveoli of the lung to the tissues. The concentration of hemoglobin within the erythrocyte and the number of erythrocytes in circulation determine how well blood will transport oxygen.

Hemoglobin consists of 4 molecules of heme, each containing 1 atom of iron, and 1 molecule of a protein, globulin. Approximately 95% of the erythrocyte dry weight is hemoglobin. Each heme/iron unit can transport 1 oxygen molecule. Therefore, each molecule of hemoglobin can carry 4 molecules of oxygen. There are over 200 million molecules of hemoglobin in each erythrocyte.

The ability of the heme molecule to carry oxygen depends on several factors. The temperature and pH of the tissues have significant effects on the oxygen-carrying capacity of hemoglobin. In the lungs, the temperature is high (equal to core temperature) and the pH is neutral. In addition, oxygen concentration is high. All these factors promote oxygenation of the hemoglobin molecule. In the peripheral tissues, the temperature, pH, and oxygen concentration are lower. In this environment, hemoglobin will release its oxygen into the tissues. The schematic in Figure 3.4 shows the mechanics of oxygen uptake and release from the erythrocyte as it travels from the lung to the tissue.

The shape of the erythrocyte also assists in delivering oxygen. In many species, the

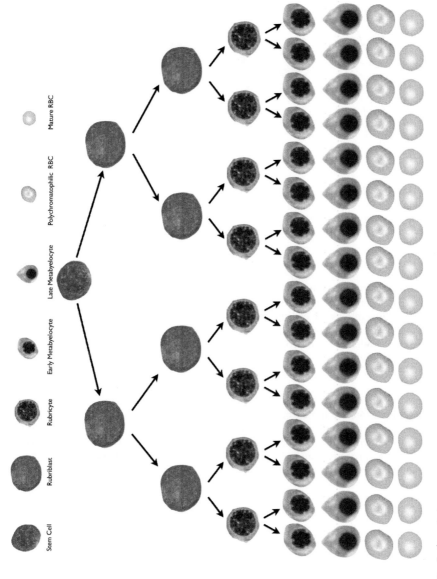

Stem Cell   Rubriblast   Rubricyte   Early Metabyelocyte   Late Metabyelocyte   Polychromatophilic RBC   Mature RBC

Figure 3.3. Erythropoiesis.

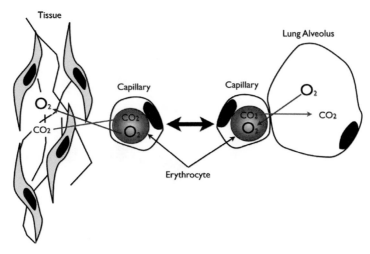

Figure 3.4. Oxygen and CO_2 transportation between the lung and the tissue. CO_2 is released from the hemoglobin in the erythrocytes in the capillary and diffuses into the lung alveolus. At the same time, oxygen diffuses from the alveolus into the capillary and is picked up by the hemoglobin in the erythrocytes. The reverse process occurs in the tissues with release of oxygen into the tissues while CO_2 is picked up by the erythrocyte for transport to the lung.

biconcave shape provides abundant surface area to exchange oxygen in the lung and tissues. The shape allows the cells to travel efficiently through the small blood vessels in the tissues (capillaries) and provides the greatest surface area possible for exchange of oxygen in the lungs and peripheral tissues.

The red cell membrane consists of protein (45%), lipid (45%), and carbohydrate (10%). Just within the membrane of the red cell is a protein "net" that maintains the shape of the erythrocyte. Figure 3.5 illustrates the membrane and protein structure of the erythrocyte.

Alterations in the lipid content of the cell's membrane or the protein net will result in changes in the erythrocyte shape. There are genetic and metabolic diseases that produce abnormal erythrocytes due to alterations in the erythrocyte membrane. For example, hereditary **elliptocytosis** is a genetic disease due to a defect in one of the network proteins in which the cells are oval-shaped rather than the normal biconcave disc.

There are many factors that affect the production of normal erythrocytes. Two processes, hemoglobin synthesis and DNA synthesis, are essential. The concentration of hemoglobin within the cytoplasm of the erythrocyte affects the division of the red cell as it matures. The maximum amount of hemoglobin in the erythrocytes is very closely regulated. Although the erythrocyte can have less hemoglobin than normal, it cannot contain a higher concentration than normal. Once the concentration of hemoglobin reaches a critical level, cell division will cease and the nucleus of the immature erythrocyte is extruded. Normal DNA synthesis is required for cell division to occur. Any process that inhibits DNA synthesis will result in decreased erythropoiesis or production of abnormal erythrocytes.

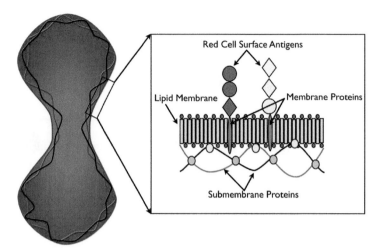

Figure 3.5. The erythrocyte shape is maintained by the protein and lipid content of the membrane and a specialized network of proteins. Any change in these structural molecules will alter the shape, and, possibly, the flexibility of the erythrocyte. Anchored in the membrane are many surface antigens that make up the blood group types.

Mammalian erythrocytes vary considerably in size and shape from species to species (Figure 3.6).

Erythrocytes depend on glucose for their energy needs (**glycolysis**). As a result, if red cells are left in contact with serum, they will continue to use glucose resulting in an artifactual decrease in serum glucose.

There are several genetic disorders of erythrocyte metabolism that result in anemia. Although relatively rare, they have been reported in several species. In most cases,

species	RBC count	Morphology	PCV	MCV	MCHC
DOG	5.5-8.5		37-55	60-77	32-36
CAT	5.0-10.0		24-45	39-55	30-36
COW	5.0-10.0		24-46	40-60	30-36
SHEEP	8.0-16.0		24-50	23-48	31-38
GOAT	8.0-18.0		19-38	15-30	35-42
HORSE	6.5-12.5		32-52	34-58	31-37

Figure 3.6. The shape, size, and number of erythrocytes varies considerably between species. The MCHC, however, is fairly similar between species.

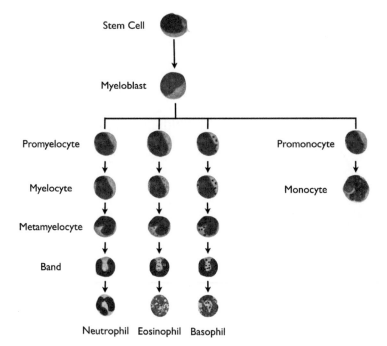

Figure 3.7.   Granulopoiesis.

the diseases are associated with hemolytic anemia.

Granulopoiesis

As with erythrocytes, circulating leukocytes are also formed in the sinusoids of the bone marrow. The progression from committed stem cells to mature leukocytes is illustrated in Figure 3.7.

Under the influence of specific growth factors, the multipotential myeloid stem cell will be committed to becoming granulocytes (i.e., neutrophils, eosinophils, basophils) or monocytes. Production of granulocytes to maintain normal numbers in the peripheral blood is a balance between stimulating growth factors and a negative feedback from the mature granulocytes in the peripheral blood. The type of granules present in their cytoplasm determines the identity of the granulocytic precursor cells.

Neutrophils

The **neutrophil** is the most common granulocyte in the peripheral blood of dogs, cats, humans, and horses. The neutrophil's name is derived from the fact that when stained with the routine **Romanowsky stains** used for peripheral blood films, the granules in their cytoplasm are "neutral"; they don't stain red (eosinophilic) or purple (basophilic). The primary function of the neutrophil is defense against bacterial disease. The neutrophil is very efficient at engulfing and destroying bacteria. The granules contain enzymes and antibacterial substances to kill and degrade bacteria. One of the most active agents within the neutrophil granule is **elastase**, an enzyme that breaks down tissue. Unfortunately, in the fulfillment of their function, they often cause significant tissue damage. A common example of this is the subcutaneous abscess.

Neutrophil Dynamics

Changes in the number of neutrophils, either increased number (**neutrophilia**) or decreased number (**neutropenia**), are the most common changes seen in the leukogram. Understanding the dynamics that determine the number of neutrophils that circulate will allow the veterinary technician to access the blood film and relate the changes to the patient. The number of circulating neutrophils depends on four separate pools of cells: proliferation pool, maturation/storage pool, circulating pool, and marginated pool. Each of these pools responds to circulating factors that can increase or decrease the number of cells in the pool population.

The Proliferation pool contains all precursors that are capable of division (stem cell, myeloblast, promyelocyte, myelocyte). The maturation and storage pool contain the postdivision neutrophils (metamelocyte, band neutrophils, mature neutrophil). In the normal animal, neutrophils are retained in this pool until they are mature and stored for quick release under the stimulation of products of inflammation. The size of the storage pool differs between species. Dogs and cats have a large storage pool; ruminants have a small storage pool and do not have the same capacity to release large numbers of mature neutrophils when needed. The most common changes in the neutrophil pools are in response to stress, excitement, and inflammation.

In response to inflammation, there is immediate release of mature neutrophils from the storage pool into the circulation. In addition, the demand for neutrophils will stimulate the proliferation pool to increase production of neutrophils for the maturation and storage pool. If the inflammatory stimulus is strong enough, immature neutrophils (band neutrophils, metamyelocytes) will be released from the maturation pool resulting in a "left shift," defined as the presence of immature neutrophils in the circulation. Occasionally, the demand for neutrophils can be so strong that it overwhelms the bone marrow, producing a **"noncompensated" left shift**. The types of neutrophil responses are discussed in Chapter 4.

In response to chronic stress with increased circulating corticosteroids, there are increased circulating neutrophils. The neutrophilia of the stress leukogram is the result of increased release of neutrophils from the storage pool and release of neutrophils from the marginated pool. The steps necessary for a neutrophil to leave circulation and migrate into the marginated pool require expression of adhesion molecules on the cells that line the capillaries (endothelial cells) and the membrane of the neutrophils. The neutrophil tumbles along the wall of the vessel until it finally adheres to the endothelial cell, and then the cell can migrate between endothelial cells into the tissues when needed. Steroids decrease the expression of receptors on the surface of the neutrophil that are responsible for adhesion of the neutrophil to the vessel wall. As a result, fewer neutrophils will be attached to the wall of the vessels decreasing the marginated pool and increasing the circulating pool.

Another common cause of neutrophilia is excitement. In this case, increased rate of blood flow in response to secretion of epinephrine "washes" neutrophils from the marginated pool into the circulating pool. In addition to the increase in neutrophils, lymphocytes also increase in response to increased release of epinephrine. In many cases, the number of lymphocytes will be greater than the neutrophils. Young dogs and cats have the most prominent excitement response.

Eosinophils

The eosinophil has eosinophilic (red) granules. Their function is not as well defined as the neutrophil's function. They are involved in response to parasitic infections, fungal disease, some protozoal diseases, allergies, and immune-complex disease. Their granules contain one of the most caustic substances found in granulocytic cells, major basic protein. This protein is thought to be responsible for the remarkable degree of necrosis found in tissues with eosinophilic inflammation. In the normal animal, very few eosinophils are present in the peripheral blood.

Basophils

The basophil has deep purple (basophilic) granules in most species and light lavender granules in the cat. Very little is known about the function of basophils. The contents of the granules are similar to those found in the mast cell, a tissue mononuclear cell that is often associated with certain inflammatory responses and allergic conditions. In normal animals, basophils are extremely rare in peripheral blood. Their number often increases in response to the same disease processes as the eosinophil.

Monocytes

The peripheral blood monocyte's primary function is to migrate to the tissues to become a macrophage. Once in the tissues, these cells participate in tissue repair, regulation of the immune response, erythrocyte turnover, and iron recycling in the spleen. They are very active cells. Monocytes circulate in relatively low numbers in the normal animal. Their numbers increase in chronic inflammatory disease and with stress in the dog. The monocyte is often confused with toxic bands and metamyelocytes. They are larger and usually have discrete vacuoles. Their nucleus is more pleomorphic (many different shapes) unlike the band neutrophil and metamyelocyte, which have distinct shapes. Figure 3.8 illustrates a monocyte compared to a band neutrophil and metamyelocyte.

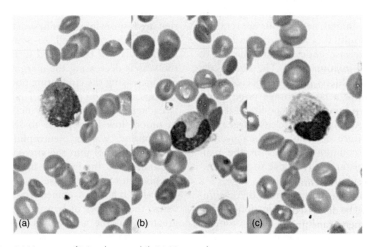

Figure 3.8.   **(a)** Monocyte. **(b)** Band neutrophil. **(c)** Metamyelocytes.

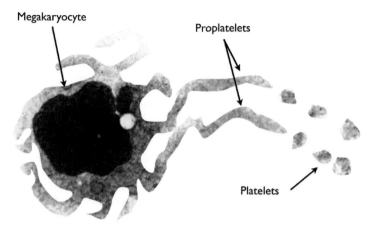

Megakaryocyte

Proplatelets

Platelets

Figure 3.9. Megakaryopoiesis. Platelets are small cytoplasmic fragments that are released from the ends of long cytoplasmic extensions (proplatelets) from the body of the megakaryocyte.

Megakaryopoiesis

Megakaryopoiesis is the production of platelets. Platelets are small fragments of megakaryocyte cytoplasm that break off of the tips of long cytoplasmic extensions called proplatelets. The production of platelets is regulated by the growth factor, **thrombopoietin**, in concert with other cytokines, some of which are part of the inflammatory process. In addition, erythropoietin can potentiate the activity of thrombopoietin. As a result of this interaction of erythropoietin and inflammatory cytokines, increased numbers of circulating platelets (**thrombocytosis**) are seen with anemia and inflammation.

Megakaryocytes are the largest cells in the bone marrow. They have large lobulated nuclei and abundant lightly granular basophilic cytoplasm. Figure 3.9 illustrates the process of platelet production.

Platelets are essential for normal blood clotting (coagulation). The process of coagulation will be discussed in Chapter 15. The platelet's membrane and cytoplasmic granules both participate in formation of blood clots. There are two types of platelet granules: dense granules and alpha-granules. Dense granules contain calcium, an essential component for the activation of clotting factors. Alpha-granules contain clotting factors and other components that promote coagulation.

Lymphocytopoiesis

The **lymphocyte** is the second most common cell type in the peripheral blood of the dog, cat, horse, and human. In the ruminant, however, the lymphocyte is the most common peripheral blood leukocyte. The primary function of the lymphocyte is to participate in acquired immunity. There are two primary types of lymphocytes: the B-cell, responsible for the production of antibodies (immunoglobulins); and the T-cell, responsible for regulation of the immune response and a process called cell-mediated immunity. The type of lymphocyte cannot be determined by its morphology. Special stains are needed to differentiate the type of lymphocyte. The morphology of the lymphocyte can change when foreign antigens stimulate the cells. Once the cells are stimulated, they become larger and develop deeply basophilic cytoplasm. Their nuclei often develop a prominent nucleolus.

Lymphocytes, initially produced in the bone marrow, migrate to several other lymphoid organs (the spleen, lymph nodes, thymus, and specific areas in the lungs and intestine) where they organize to form the lymphoid system. The lymphocytes present in the peripheral blood circulate into and out of these lymphoid organs as they survey the body for foreign antigens or infectious agents. Lymphoid cells that leave the peripheral blood are returned to circulation through the lymphatic vessels that arise in the tissues and eventually are dumped into the vena cava through the thoracic duct in the thoracic cavity. Figure 3.10 illustrates the organs involved in the lymphoid system.

The thymus is the source of T-cells. The environment of the thymus allows the body to identify lymphocytes that have the potential to react to the individual's own tissue and remove them from the body

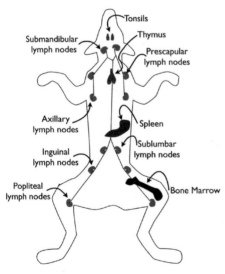

Figure 3.10. An illustration of lymph nodes and lymph flow through the canine body.

while keeping lymphocytes that will not react to self. This allows the body to identify nonself antigens from foreign bacteria and pathogens while not attacking the body's own tissue. The thymus and the bone marrow are the two lymphoid organs that can produce lymphocytes without immune stimulation. Over time, the thymus decreases in size and function by a process called involution. The remaining lymphoid organs produce lymphocytes when stimulated by a foreign antigen.

The spleen is a large vascular organ with two primary functions. It is the largest secondary lymphoid organ and acts as a blood filter. The tissue of the spleen has two distinct regions, the red and white pulp. The name for these regions comes from the fact that on cut surface, small round white spots corresponding to the lymphoid tissue (white pulp) are scattered throughout the highly vascular red pulp. The filtering function of the spleen allows it to remove abnormal erythrocytes. As blood flows through the sinusoids of the spleen through the red pulp, old, atypically shaped, parasitized, immune-injured, and nucleated erythrocytes are removed. In addition, the spleen's lymphoid tissue, the white pulp, continually surveys the blood as it passes through its vessels and sinusoids for foreign antigens.

The lymph nodes are small, bean-shaped organs that filter lymph and transport lymphocytes and other cells from the tissues back to the blood. Lymph is fluid from the tissues that is collected in specialized thin-walled vessels, the **lymphatics**; filtered through the lymph nodes; and finally returned to the blood through the thoracic duct, which empties into the vena cava within the thorax. Multiple lymphatic vessels enter a lymph node through its capsule and exit through a single vessel. The lymph percolates through the cortex to the medulla of the lymph node exposing the resident lymphocytes to all components in the fluid.

Abnormalities in the Red and White Blood Cell Populations

It is much easier to understand changes that occur in response to disease when one has a strong understanding of normal blood and blood cells. This chapter reviews common changes in the hemogram associated with disease. Changes in erythrocyte and leukocyte morphology and their underlying causes are discussed, and the pathogenesis (steps involved in the development of a disease) of anemia, polycythemia, leukocytosis, leukopenia, thrombocytosis, and thrombocytopenia are described along with the diseases that are associated with these abnormal hemogram findings.

Abnormalities in Erythrocyte Morphology

Changes in the morphology of erythrocytes include changes in shape and inclusions in or on the erythrocyte. Each of these morphological abnormalities provides information about disease processes that may be present. Several erythrocyte abnormalities provide an insight into the underlying cause for anemia or prompt the close evaluation of the functions of certain organs, such as the liver, spleen, and kidney. Recognition of these morphological changes is an essential skill for veterinary technicians who review blood films.

Poikilocytes

Erythrocyte morphology has its own language, as do many areas of medicine. Poikilocytosis simply indicates that the red blood cells seen on review of a blood film have abnormal shapes. There are several specific shape changes that warrant identification to assist the clinician in interpreting changes in the hemogram. Poikilocytes are abnormally shaped erythrocytes. The most common types of poikilocytes are echinocytes (crenated erythrocytes), acanthocytes, schistocytes, spherocytes, keratocytes, burr cells, eccentrocytes, and target cells. Less common poikilocytes include stomatocytes and ovalocytes. Figure 4.1

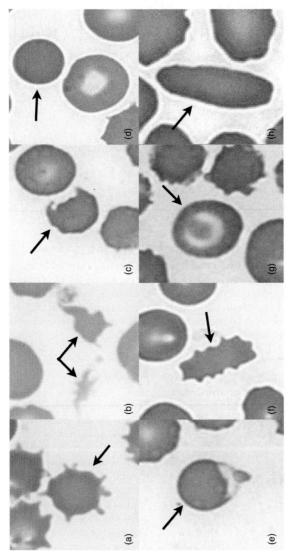

Figure 4.1. (a) acanthocyte. (b) schistocyte. (c) Keratocyte. (d) spherocyte. (e) eccentrocyte. (f) ovaloechinocyte (burr cell). (g) torocyte (target cell). (h) Ovalocyte.

Table 4.1.   Common poikilocytosis and associated diseases.

Type of Cell Noted	Shape of Cell	Disease
Echinocytes (crenated cell)	Numerous uniformly distributed tent-shaped spikes	Artifact of drying, snake bite, dehydration, inherited erythrocyte defects
Acanthocytes	Irregularly spaced thin spikes with knoblike tips; no central pallor	Prominent numbers: liver disease, renal disease, hemangiosarcoma Small numbers: iron deficiency, microangiopathy
Eccentrocytes	Dense eccentric displacement of hemoglobin with a clear edge	Oxidative injury secondary to onion toxicity, drugs
Schistocytes	Small irregular fragments of the erythrocyte	Microangiopathy, iron deficiency, hemangiosarcoma, valvular stenosis
Spherocytes	Small dense cells with no central pallor	Large numbers: hemolytic anemia Small numbers: microangiopathy, iron deficiency
Keratocytes	Surface blisters that rupture to form small hornlike extensions.	Iron deficiency, microangiopathy, liver disease
Burr cells (ovalo-echinocytes)	Elongate cells with spikes similar to a crenated cell	Feline liver disease, renal disease

illustrates each of the most common types of poikilocytes. Crenated cells, target cells, and stomatocytes can be seen as artifacts of drying as well as in association with a disease process. Table 4.1 lists the common poikilocytes and disease associated with each shape.

Echinocytes are erythrocytes with spiky protrusions from their surface. They are the most common poikilocytes seen on blood films. There are several types of echinocytes; **crenated cells** and **acanthocytes** are the most commonly seen. Crenated erythrocytes can be seen on blood films as an artifact when the blood film dries slowly. Crenation can also be seen in dehydrated animals and secondary to snake bite. Crenated cells have regularly placed tent-shaped projections from their surface. They also retain a central area of light staining, central pallor, characteristic of the normal discoid shape of the red blood cell. A useful test to determine whether the crenation is an artifact or true

shape change is to view a wet-mount preparation of the blood. One drop of blood and two drops of saline can be mixed on a glass slide, coverslipped, and viewed on the microscope. True crenation will still be present when viewed on the wet-mount preparation.

Unlike crenated cells, **acanthocytes** are not associated with artifact but are considered true morphological changes when seen on the blood film. They differ from crenated cells in several ways. The projections present on acanthocytes are irregularly placed, they have variable-sized knobs on the tips of the spiky projections, and they generally do not retain an area of central pallor. Acanthocytes are associated with several disease processes. Renal disease, liver disease, iron deficiency, microangiopathy (formation of small fibrin clots in capillaries), and vascular neoplasia (hemangiosarcoma) are the most common causes of acanthocytosis in veterinary patients. The exact mechanism of acanthocyte formation in veterinary patients is not fully understood. It is thought to be due to changes in membrane lipids that make the cells more rigid and prone to deformation as they circulate through capillaries. When acanthocytes are seen on the blood film, it should prompt the clinician to further evaluate the liver, spleen, and kidneys for possible dysfunction.

Spherocytes are small erythrocytes with no central pallor. Spherocytes are a hallmark of immune-mediated hemolytic anemia, but they can also be seen in small numbers in association with other types of erythrocyte damage. Spherocytes are formed when a macrophage removes an abnormal portion of the erythrocyte membrane, causing the erythrocyte to form a sphere instead of the normal biconcave disc (partial phagocytosis) (Figure 4.2).

The biconcave disc shape of the normal erythrocyte cannot be maintained if a portion of the membrane is lost. Spherocytes are easier to see in canine blood than in feline blood because of the normal shape of the erythrocyte in these two species. The dog has a more pronounced central pallor compared to the smaller erythrocyte with much less central pallor in the cat. Accurate identification of spherocytes requires the evaluation of erythrocytes in the counting area only. Erythrocytes at the feathered edge do not have an area of central pallor. There will usually be normal erythrocytes to compare to the spherocyte in the counting area. The spherocyte will appear small and dense. In addition to immune-mediated mechanisms, spherocytes can be seen with erythrocyte fragmentation (discussed below). In most cases, a high number of spherocytes in an anemic patient with no other erythrocyte morphological changes is indicative of immune-mediated hemolysis.

Spherocytes can also be seen with hypersplenism, a splenic disease in which the spleen removes excessive numbers of erythrocytes due to abnormal macrophage

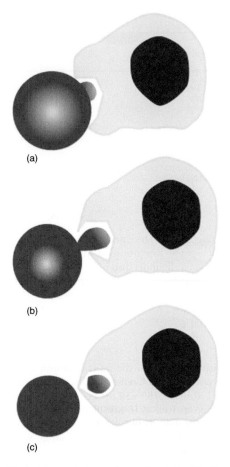

(a)

(b)

(c)

Figure 4.2. Formation of a spherocyte. **(a)** The macrophage recognizes a defect in the membrane of a red cell and begins the process of partial phagocytosis. **(b)** The macrophages "pinches off' the abnormal portion of the red cell membrane. **(c)** The remaining red cell membrane cannot maintain the normal biconcave shape, and the red cell becomes a sphere that is smaller than the original red cell and has no central pallor.

function. Spherocytes associated with additional erythrocyte changes (schistocytes, acanthocytes, keratocytes) indicate nonimmune mechanisms of spherocyte formation. The nonimmune causes of spherocyte formation include toxins such as zinc and copper as well as hypophosphatemia (see

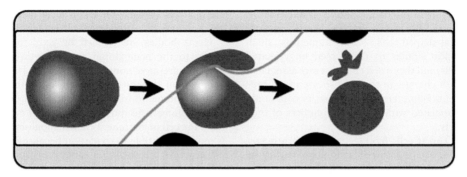

Figure 4.3. Formation of a schistocyte. The red cell encounters a fibrin strand, and a small portion of the cell membrane is cut from the cell forming a spherocyte and a small fragment (schistocyte).

Chapter 8). The mechanisms underlying spherocyte formation in these conditions is not well understood, but it may relate to oxidative injury to the membrane with formation of hemoglobin crystals in the erythrocyte membrane (**Heinz bodies**) and partial phagocytosis of the erythrocyte by macrophages.

Schistocytes are small fragments of erythrocytes that are irregular in size and shape. This erythrocyte change is a hallmark of erythrocyte fragmentation. The erythrocytes are fragmented as they circulate through abnormal capillaries or tortuous vascular channels present in some forms of neoplasia. One of the most common causes of schistocyte formation is **microangiopathy**. Microangiopathy is a consequence of many diseases. Microangiopathy is essentially the formation of fibrin strands or small fibrin clots within capillaries and is associated with disseminated intravascular coagulation. The syndrome of **disseminated intravascular coagulation** and its causes is fully discussed in Chapter 13. Schistocytes are often seen concurrently with small numbers of spherocytes, acanthocytes, and keratocytes. Figure 4.3 illustrates the fragmentation of an erythrocyte as it passes through a capillary that contains fibrin strands with formation of a schistocyte and a spherocyte. Turbulent blood

flow associated with abnormal blood vessels, abnormal heart valves (valvular stenosis), vascular neoplasia, and obstructions to blood flow (severe heartworm disease) can also cause formation of schistocytes. Intrinsic changes to the erythrocyte membrane that increase cell fragility will also result in fragmentation (e.g., iron deficiency and doxorubicin toxicity).

Eccentrocytes are erythrocytes with fusion of a portion of the cell membrane that causes the hemoglobin to be pushed to the side. Oxidative injury to the erythrocyte is the cause of the fusion. This morphological change is seen most commonly in the dog. The most common cause of eccentrocyte formation in the dog is onion toxicity. Zinc toxicity can also result in eccentrocyte formation in the dog. Heinz bodies, another erythrocyte abnormality associated with oxidative injury, are usually present along with eccentrocyte. Both eccentrocytes and erythrocytes with Heinz bodies will have a shorter half-life and an increased chance of being removed from circulation by the macrophages of the spleen.

Keratocytes and **burr cells** are erythrocyte morphological changes associated with many different erythrocyte abnormalities. Keratocytes are erythrocytes that have small "blisters" on their surface that rupture. Keratocytes can be seen with increased fragility, microangiopathy, and oxidative injury. Burr cells (ovalo-echinocytes) are oval-shaped cells with numerous small spikes similar to those seen on crenated cells, and they are seen in diseases associated with changes in the erythrocyte membrane lipid. Feline hepatic lipidosis is commonly associated with increased numbers of burr cells.

Target cells (codocytes) are erythrocytes with a central area of hemoglobin within the area of central pallor forming a target appearance. Target cells are usually an artifact of drying. They can be seen with regenerative anemia, liver disease, endocrine disease (hypothyroidism), and iron deficiency. The target appearance is thought to be due to the fact that the cells have excessive membrane for their volume and are "floppy."

Erythrocyte Inclusions

In addition to poikilocytosis, erythrocytes can contain a variety of abnormal structures (inclusions) that are associated with certain disease processes. Heinz bodies, Howell-Jolly bodies, and basophilic stippling are the most common inclusions. Figure 4.4 illustrates the common noninfectious inclusions found in erythrocytes. Erythroparasites (parasitic diseases of the erythrocyte)

are also associated with erythrocyte inclusions and are discussed later in this chapter.

Heinz bodies are formed by oxidative injury to the hemoglobin in the erythrocyte and are most common in the cat. The hemoglobin denatures and adheres to the cell membrane, forming a spherical light or clear staining inclusion that may extend out from the cell membrane. Feline hemoglobin is more susceptible to oxidation because of its structure. Hemoglobin molecules from different species have variable numbers of sulfhydryl groups (composed of sulfur and hydrogen). These groups are very susceptible to oxidation and the more sulfhydryl groups a molecule of hemoglobin has, the more likely Heinz bodies will form when the patient undergoes oxidative stress. Feline hemoglobin has twice the number of sulfhydryl groups per molecule than dog hemoglobin.

Heinz body formation is associated with anemia because the spleen will remove erythrocytes with Heinz bodies. The most common causes for Heinz body formation in the cat are toxic (acetaminophen, propylene glycol, propofol) and metabolic (diabetes mellitus, renal disease, lymphoma, hyperthyroidism). The less common causes of Heinz body anemia include methylene blue, vitamin K3, benzocaine products, phenols, d-L methionine, phenazopyridine, naphthalene, zinc, and copper.

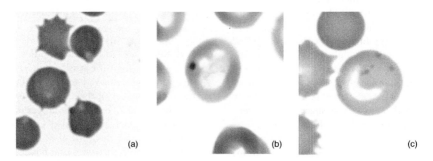

(a)   (b)   (c)

Figure 4.4. Common inclusions in erythrocytes. **(a)** Heinz bodies. **(b)** Howell-Jolly body. **(c)** Basophilic stippling.

A good drug history is essential in determining the underlying cause of a Heinz body anemia. Heinz bodies can be large or small and difficult to identify. Large Heinz bodies are more easily identified because they project out from the surface of the erythrocyte. Smaller Heinz bodies are more difficult to find because they are seen as small lightly staining areas within the erythrocyte. The smaller Heinz bodies are present in small numbers in normal feline blood and may increase in number in cats with metabolic disease. The smaller Heinz body may not be associated with anemia, and significant numbers of large Heinz bodies are usually associated with anemia.

Howell-Jolly bodies are small remnants of the erythrocyte nucleus that occasionally remain after the nucleus undergoes division. These small fragments may not be extruded with the nucleus as the erythrocyte matures. In the normal state, erythrocytes with Howell-Jolly bodies will be removed by the spleen. Splenectomy and any condition that inhibits normal splenic function (increased circulating corticosteroids, septicemia/endotoxemia, hypoxia) will result in increased numbers of circulating erythrocytes with Howell-Jolly bodies. When erythrocyte production is accelerated, more erythrocytes will have Howell-Jolly bodies when released into circulation. Cats normally tend to have a few erythrocytes with Howell-Jolly bodies because their spleen is not as efficient at removing abnormal erythrocytes. The unique filtering capability of the feline spleen also contributes to the fact that cats often have more circulating Heinz bodies than the dog.

Basophilic stippling of erythrocytes is characterized by fine basophilic reticulum that is seen on Wright-Giemsa stains. The reticulum is aggregated RNA (just as in reticulocytes) and is occasionally seen in regenerative anemia. When basophilic stippling is seen in a regenerative anemia, it is usually found in young polychromatophilic erythrocytes. Basophilic stippling can also be seen with lead poisoning.

Siderocytes are erythrocytes with iron-containing basophilic inclusions. They are relatively uncommon but can be seen in patients with erythrocyte destruction and increased erythrocyte turnover rate.

Anemia

Anemia, a decreased number of red blood cells as measured by the PCV/Hct, is one of the most common abnormalities seen in the CBC of an ill patient. Clinical signs suggestive of anemia include pale mucous membranes, increased respiratory rate, and, in some cases, icterus (yellow coloration of tissues). The initial step in evaluating an anemic patient is to determine whether the patient's bone marrow can increase production of erythrocytes in response to the decrease in PCV. The presence of a bone marrow response separates anemia into two broad categories, regenerative and nonregenerative. A regenerative anemia is defined as an anemia with evidence that the bone marrow can respond by increased production of erythrocyte. Erythropoietin, the hormone released by the kidneys in response to the decrease in oxygen-carrying capacity of the blood, is the stimulus for the bone marrow to increase production of erythrocytes. A regenerative anemia indicates that the patient has a normal functioning bone marrow and normal production of erythropoietin by the kidney interstitium. A nonregenerative anemia is defined as an anemia with no evidence that the bone marrow can respond. The lack of response by the bone marrow can be due to a disease that directly affects the bone marrow or decreased production of erythropoietin by the kidney, usually due to chronic renal failure. Table 4.2 lists the more common causes of regenerative and nonregenerative anemias.

Table 4.2.   Causes of regenerative and nonregenerative anemia.

Regenerative Anemia	Nonregenerative Anemia
Blood loss (trauma, coagulation defects)	Bone marrow neoplasia (leukemia, nonmarrow [metastatic])
Immune-mediated hemolytic anemia	Bone marrow fibrosis
Oxidative hemolytic anemia	Infectious disease (FeLV, chronic ehrlichiosis)
Erythroparasites	Toxicity
	Chronic renal disease (lack of erythropoietin)

Regenerative Anemia

The classification of an anemia as regenerative is based on identifying several changes found in the hemogram and on the blood film that are indicative of release of young erythrocytes (polychromatophilic red blood cells). Young erythrocytes produced in response to anemia are larger than normal because they are produced more rapidly and released sooner than normal. When significant numbers of these large polychromatophilic cells are present in circulation, the mean cell volume (MCV) will increase and if there are a sufficient number of them, the MCV will be above the reference range indicating macrocytosis (large erythrocytes). The larger polychromatophilic cells have a lower concentration of hemoglobin compared to normal erythrocytes because they usually contain the same amount of hemoglobin in a larger volume. As a result, the mean cell hemoglobin concentration (MCHC) will be decreased indicating **hypochromasia** (cells with decreased staining of their cytoplasm). Figure 4.5 shows a photomicrograph illustrating hypochromasia and macrocytosis.

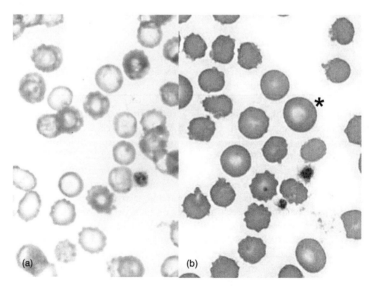

Figure 4.5.   **(a)** Hypochromasia. **(b)** Macrocytosis.

A high MCV and low MCHC are excellent indicators of regeneration, but they cannot be used as the sole indication of regeneration. There are few instances where the MCV may be misleading when evaluating an anemic patient. Small populations of poodles and Akitas have MCV values that are out of the reference range for most dogs. Individual poodles may have a genetic trait (**poodle macrocytosis**) that results in a normal MCV higher than other dogs (100 fl compared to 60–77 fl for most dogs). A subpopulation of Akitas, and perhaps other Japanese breeds, has erythrocytes that are significantly smaller than other dogs (45 fl compared to 60–77 fl for most dogs). In the first case, a poodle with a nonregenerative anemia may be thought to have a regenerative anemia because its MCV is high, even though it is normal for that individual dog. In the second case, an Akita with a regenerative anemia may be considered to have a nonregenerative anemia because its MCV is within the reference range for other dogs, even though it is increased for that individual. In the cat, FeLV infection can cause a nonregenerative macrocytic anemia with a remarkably high MCV in the face of severe bone marrow dysfunction.

As a result of these exceptions and because the degree of macrocytosis and hypochromasia is an insensitive indicator of regeneration, review of the blood film and a reticulocyte count are necessary to confirm a regenerative response. The presence of polychromatophic cells on the blood film is required in order to confirm regeneration, and an increased reticulocyte count is necessary to determine whether the regenerative response is sufficient for the degree of anemia.

Polychromatophilic erythrocytes are usually larger than normal erythrocytes, and they have a larger central pallor and a blue hue when stained with Wright-Giemsa stain and a muddy blue hue when stained with Diff-Quik Wright-Giemsa™. A standard method of reporting the amount of poly-

Table 4.3. Semiquantitation method for polychromasia.

Degree of Polychromasia	Number of Polychromatophilic Cells/1000×
few	0–1
1+	1–2 (dog), 0–1 (cat)
2+	2–3 (dog), 1–2 (cat)
3+	3–6 (dog), 2–4 (cat)
4+	6 (dog), >4 (cat)

chromasia should be used when evaluating the blood film for evidence of a regenerative anemia. Table 4.3 shows a common method for reporting degree of polychromasia based on number of polychromatic cells seen per 1000× field. Reporting polychromasia is a subjective method and is not as accurate as counting the number of reticulocytes/1000 cells using a reticulocyte stain. Reticulocyte stains are stains that precipitate residual RNA in the erythrocytes and stain the precipitate dark blue. Young erythrocytes have more residual RNA than mature erythrocytes and will stain with a distinct blue "reticulum"—hence the name reticulocyte. There are two types of reticulocytes, aggregate and punctate. Dogs have aggregate reticulocytes only. Cats have both punctate and aggregate forms. Figure 4.6 illustrates reticulocyte stain preparations from a dog and a cat.

Reticulocyte counts are not difficult to perform; however, they do require patience. Unlike other blood film stains, reticulocyte stains are added to the blood before the blood film preparation is made. When using new methylene blue, 5 drops of whole blood and 5 drops of a 0.5% solution of new methylene blue are mixed in a small tube and allowed to sit for 5 to 10 minutes, after which a blood film is prepared. A reticulocyte count is done by counting the number of reticulocytes found while examining

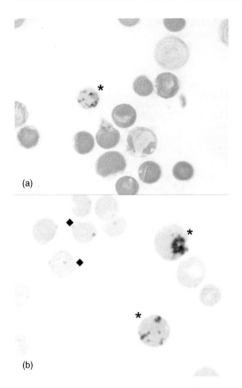

(a)

(b)

Figure 4.6.   Reticulocyte stains. **(a)** Dog. **(b)** Cat. Note the aggregate (∗) and the punctate (◇) reticulocytes in the cat.

1000 erythrocytes. This is time consuming and is usually done at a reference laboratory. In addition, newer large hematology instruments used by reference laboratories can accurately count reticulocytes as part of the automated CBC.

A close estimate of the reticulocyte count, which is fairly accurate, can be done in the clinic. In the area of the blood film where the erythrocytes are touching or just overlapping, the number of erythrocytes in a standard 1000× field is approximately 200 cells for the dog and slightly more for the cat. Counting the number of reticulocytes in five of these fields will provide a good estimate of the number of reticulocytes/1000 erythrocytes. This number is then divided

by 10 to obtain the percentage of reticulocytes in the erythrocyte population. As with all methods used to estimate a value from the blood film, a quick low-power scan of the blood film is necessary to ensure that there is an even distribution of reticulocytes in the area to be counted. This method can be validated in the clinic by comparing the estimated count to that obtained at a reference laboratory on the same blood sample.

The number of reticulocytes can be reported as a percentage or an absolute number, just as is done with leukocyte numbers. Multiplying the red blood cell count by the percentage of reticulocytes will provide an absolute number of reticulocytes. Figure 4.7 illustrates the calculation of an estimated reticulocyte count and an absolute reticulocyte count. The degree of regeneration, measured by percent reticulocytes should be greater as the degree of anemia increases if the bone marrow is working to its highest capacity. The percent reticulocyte count should be corrected for the degree of anemia by using a factor that takes into account the patient's PCV and the normal PCV of the patient's species.

Example: An anemic cat has a PCV of 18% and a 3.0% reticulocyte count. The percent reticulocyte count is corrected by multiplying the 3.0% by the patient's PCV divided by 35 (for the cat):

$$3.0\% \times 18/35 \; (35 \text{ for a cat, or } 45 \text{ for a dog}) = 1.5\%$$

The absolute number of reticulocytes does not need to be corrected because it is based on the degree of anemia (the red blood cell count). There are accepted ranges for absolute reticulocyte counts and percent reticulocytes that indicate the degree of response. Table 4.4 lists reticulocyte percentages and absolute numbers that correspond to the degree of regeneration.

In addition to polychromasia, increased numbers of **metarubricytes** (nucleated red

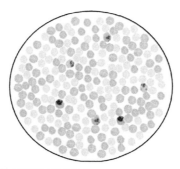

Calculating a % reticulocyte count:

1. Count the number of reticulocytes in 5 oil immersion fields in the body of reticulocyte-stained blood film.

2. Divide by 10.

Example:
        30 reticulocytes counted in 5 oil immersion fields.
        30/10 = 3.0%

Figure 4.7. Estimation of the reticulocyte percent.

blood cells (nRBC)) may be released by the marrow into the peripheral blood. The release of metarubricytes in a regenerative anemia will always be accompanied by a significant polychromatophilia and an increased reticulocyte count. This is termed an appropriate metarubricytosis. An inappropriate metarubricytosis is defined as an increased number of metarubricytes in the circulation without other evidence of regeneration. An inappropriate metarubricytosis is seen with bone marrow injury, splenectomy, lead poisoning, and neoplastic processes such as leukemia of the erythrocyte precursors. The most common causes for an inappropriate metarubricytosis are splenic disease, extramedullary hematopoiesis, and splenectomy. Other disease processes associated with inappropriate metarubricytosis are hypoxia, bone marrow necrosis, sepsis/endotoxemia, and neoplasia (splenic hemangiosarcoma). Any disease that inhibits splenic function can result in an inappropriate metarubricytosis. The macrophages of the spleen are responsible for removing abnormal erythrocytes in the peripheral blood, and metarubricytes should not be in the peripheral circulation.

Table 4.4. Reticulocyte percentages and absolute numbers and corresponding degree of regeneration.

Reticulocyte Percentage (Corrected)	Absolute Reticulocyte	Degree of Regeneration
<1% (dog), <0.4% (cat)	<60,000 (dog), <40,000 (cat)	No regeneration
1–4% (dog), 0.5–2% (cat)	60–150,000 (dog), 40–70,000 (cat)	Mild regeneration
5–20% (dog), 3–4% (cat)	150–300,000 (dog), 70–100,000(cat)	Moderate regeneration
<20% (dog), >4% (cat)	300,000 (dog), >100,000 (cat)	Marked regeneration

Corticosteroid administration will inhibit the function of splenic macrophages as well.

Regardless of the cause of the increase in metarubricytes in the peripheral blood, if they are present they will be counted by all in-house hematology instruments and in the manual WBC count as leukocytes. As a result, the leukocyte count must be corrected for the number of metarubricytes seen while doing the differential. The calculation for correcting the leukocyte count is (100/(100 + number of nRBCs counted on differential)) × WBC count.

Example: 10 nRBCs noted during the 100 cell differential count and the WBC count is 11,000/µl:

$$(100/(100 + 10)) \times 11,000/\mu l = 10,000/\mu l$$

If the leukocyte count is high enough to require a 200 cell differential then the calculation would be: (200/(200 + the number of nRBCs counted during the differential)) × WBC count.

Anemia due to Blood Loss

Once an anemia is confirmed as regenerative, the cause of the regenerative anemia must be determined. There are two general causes for a regenerative anemia, blood loss or blood destruction. Anemia due to external blood loss is associated with low total protein because protein and blood cells are both lost with bleeding. The development of anemia following a significant bleed takes approximately 4 hours. The PCV and total protein are eventually diluted by the influx of fluid into the vascular system in an attempt to replace the blood lost. As a result of this, measuring a PCV and total protein earlier than 4 hours after a potential bleeding will not reveal an anemia.

Internal blood loss into body cavities such as the thorax and abdomen results in a decrease in PCV but not total protein. The protein is reabsorbed from the body cavity while about half of the erythrocytes are recovered by the lymphatic system; the remainder of the erythrocytes either lyse or are engulfed by macrophages. The regenerative response to blood loss is usually moderate. In most cases, there is no significant red cell morphology abnormality associated with acute blood loss other than increased numbers of Howell-Jolly bodies and polychromasia.

Chronic external blood loss can be seen with gastrointestinal ulcers, ulcerated gastrointestinal neoplasms, chronic hematuria, and internal and external parasitism. Over time, chronic blood loss shifts from a regenerative anemia to a nonregenerative anemia because of loss of the iron in hemoglobin. In the normal turnover of erythrocytes, iron is recycled. If chronic blood loss has resulted in sufficient loss of iron and overwhelmed the body's ability to absorb dietary iron in sufficient quantities, iron deficiency anemia will occur. Iron deficiency anemia is associated with **microcytosis** (decreased MCV) and **hypochromasia** (decreased MCHC). The erythrocytes will appear pale with a large area of central pallor and there will be remarkable anisocytosis (variation in erythrocyte size) present on the blood film.

In addition, red cell morphology changes can be seen because of increased erythrocyte fragility associated with iron deficiency. Schistocytes, acanthocytes, and keratocytes are abnormal erythrocyte changes associated with iron deficiency. Figure 4.8 illustrates several erythrocyte changes that are associated with iron deficiency. Iron deficiency is more common and develops more rapidly in young animals, because they have limited iron in their diets if they are still nursing and their bone marrow has a smaller pool of stored iron. Adult animals usually develop iron deficiency with prolonged bleeding that is difficult to identify on physical exam, such as a bleeding gastrointestinal lesion that does not produce overt melena.

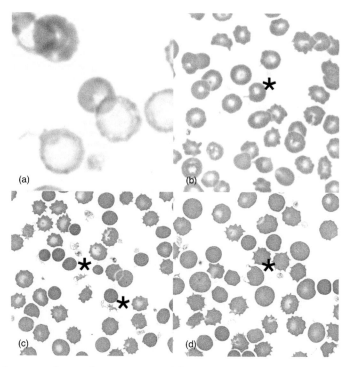

Figure 4.8. Common erythrocyte changes seen in iron deficiency. **(a)** Hypochromasia. **(b)** Budding fragmentation. **(c)** Schistocyte. **(d)** Keratocyte.

Anemia due to Blood Destruction (Hemolytic Anemia)

Hemolytic anemia can occur by several mechanisms including toxicity, erythroparasitism, and immune-mediated disease. In contrast to blood loss anemia, the total protein in hemolytic anemia is usually normal. There are two broad types of hemolytic anemia, intravascular and extravascular. Table 4.5 lists diseases associated with erythrocyte destruction and their most common mechanisms. Intravascular hemolysis is the process by which erythrocytes lyse in the blood vessel, resulting in release of their hemoglobin (**hemoglobinemia**).

Extravascular hemolysis is the process by which macrophages in the spleen and liver engulf and destroy damaged erythrocytes and break down hemoglobin to recover the iron and release bilirubin (a breakdown product of heme) into the circulation resulting in an increase in circulating bilirubin (**hyperbilirubinemia**). Many hemolytic diseases are associated with both intravascular and extravascular mechanisms. Factors that can influence the type of hemolysis include the type of antibody causing the lysis in immune-mediated disease, the severity of infection with erythroparasitism, and the severity of oxidative injury with toxicity.

Intravascular hemolysis often causes a more severe disease because of the toxic effects of free hemoglobin on the kidneys and the widespread inflammation associated with release of hemoglobin into the

Table 4.5. Diseases associated with erythrocyte destruction and mechanisms.

Immune-mediated hemolytic anemia	Extravascular hemolysis: macrophage removal of antibody-coated erythrocytes	Intravascular hemolysis: lysis of erythrocytes by antibody on the cell surface
Heinz body anemia/eccentrocyte-associated anemia	Oxidative injury to hemoglobin (zinc, drugs); extravascular hemolysis: macrophage removal of erythrocytes with Heinz bodies	
Erythroparasites	Extravascular hemolysis: macrophage removal of infected erythrocytes (antibodies to the organism contributes to the phagocytosis)	Intravascular hemolysis: lysis of heavily infected erythrocytes (may be antibody-mediated)
Hypophosphatemia	Extravascular hemolysis: removal of erythrocytes with oxidative injury	Intravascular hemolysis, possibly due to disruption of erythrocyte metabolism

blood. Hemoglobinemia is seen as a red discoloration of the serum or plasma (Figure 4.9a). When evaluating a patient with hemoglobinemia, it is very important to be sure that the hemoglobinemia is truly due to lysis of the erythrocyte within the patient's vessels. In some cases of hemolytic anemia,

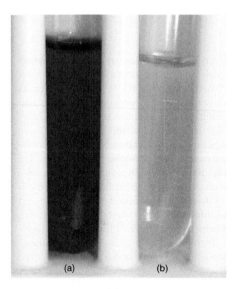

Figure 4.9. **(a)** Hemoglobinemia. **(b)** Hyperbilirubinemia (icterus).

the damaged erythrocytes are fragile but do not lyse in the vessel; they are removed by the macrophage system. However, during the process of venipuncture, the fragile cells will lyse as they are drawn into the syringe or vacutainer. One simple way to determine whether the lysis is truly intravascular is to evaluate the urine. Patients with true hemoglobinemia will have **hemoglobinuria** (red urine due to the presence of hemoglobin). When hemolysis is present, the MCHC is usually increased. This is an artifactual increase because erythrocytes cannot contain a higher concentration of hemoglobin than normal. Occasionally, an MCHC will be increased without concurrent hemoglobinemia. When this occurs, it indicates that there is some component other than hemoglobin in the blood that is being measured as hemoglobin by the instrument. The most common causes of this artifact are lipemia, Heinz bodies (denatured hemoglobin), and abnormal proteins.

Extravascular hemolysis is more common than intravascular hemolysis. When the hemolysis is severe, it is associated with hyperbilirubinemia and jaundice (yellow discoloration of the tissues). Hyperbilirubinemia, if severe enough, causes a yellow discoloration of the serum or plasma

(Figure 4.9b). The patient with extravascular hemolysis will become jaundiced when the amount of bilirubin produced overwhelms the liver's ability to excrete the bilirubin through the bile. Most forms of immune-mediated anemia are due to extravascular hemolysis. In all forms of extravascular hemolysis, there is a structural alteration in the erythrocyte that triggers phagocytosis by macrophages in the spleen and liver. Antibodies, parasites, hemoglobin crystals, and fused membranes are the most common erythrocyte structural changes associated with increased erythrocyte removal by macrophages.

There are several changes in the peripheral blood that can assist in the diagnosis of hemolytic anemia and help identify the underlying cause of the hemolysis. One of the most striking examples is visible agglutination of erythrocytes seen with immune-mediated hemolytic anemia. Marked agglutination (clumping of erythrocytes due to immune mechanisms) is seen as large red "flakes" in the sample as it is rotated (Figure 4.10a). On the blood film, the clusters of agglutinated erythrocytes are seen throughout the blood film, most prominently at the feathered edge. In some cases, the agglutination is so severe that it is impossible to make a good blood film (Figure 4.10b). When agglutination is seen, it is important to be sure that it is true agglutination caused by antibodies linking the erythrocytes together and not a nonspecific "stickiness" caused by inflammatory proteins in the plasma. The saline agglutination test is very useful in differentiating these two causes of erythrocyte clumping.

Use the following steps for the saline agglutination test method:

1. Add 5 drops of blood to 2 ml of saline and mix gently.
2. Centrifuge the sample on the same setting as a urine sample.
3. Pour off supernatant, add an additional 2 ml of saline and mix gently.

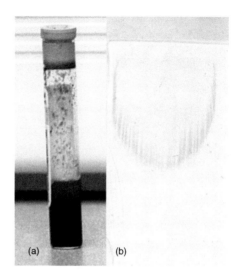

Figure 4.10. **(a)** EDTA tube showing gross agglutination. **(b)** Blood film showing a "reverse" feather edge due to marked erythrocyte agglutination.

4. Centrifuge a second time.
5. Pour off supernatant and resuspend the erythrocyte pellet in 2 ml of saline.
6. Prepare a wet-mount of the cell suspension by placing 2 drops of the suspension on a glass slide and cover with a coverslip; evaluate on low power.

Figure 4.11 shows the results of a positive and a negative saline agglutination test. One of the most common abnormalities associated with immune-mediated hemolytic anemia is the presence of significant numbers of spherocytes. Other forms of hemolytic anemia are associated with toxicities resulting in oxidative injury with formation of Heinz bodies and eccentrocytes (e.g., acetaminophen, zinc toxicity, copper toxicity, hypophosphatemia) and erythroparasitism. There are hereditary hemolytic anemias associated with both erythrocyte structural abnormalities and enzyme deficiencies. Table 4.6 provides a list of hereditary diseases of the erythrocyte that result in hemolytic anemia.

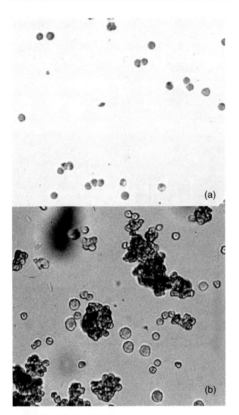

Figure 4.11. Saline agglutination test. **(a)** Negative for true agglutination. **(b)** Positive for true agglutination.

Table 4.6. Hereditary diseases associated with hemolytic anemia.

Disease	Common Breed
Hereditary spherocytosis	Miniature schnauzers, Alaskan malamutes
Pyruvate kinase deficiency	Basenji, beagles, West Highland white terriers, cairn terriers, miniature poodles
Phosphofructokinase deficiency	English springer spaniels, American cocker spaniel

Nonregenerative Anemia

Nonregenerative anemia occurs when the bone marrow cannot continue to replace erythrocytes that are removed due to aging. This includes diseases that directly affect the bone marrow and non–bone marrow diseases that can inhibit the bone marrow. In nonregenerative anemia, the bone marrow cannot produce new erythrocytes in sufficient numbers to maintain a normal PCV/Hct. Primary bone marrow failure is seen with toxins, neoplasia, and, rarely, with nutritional causes. In addition, there are poorly understood primary bone marrow diseases such as **aplastic anemia** and pure red cell aplasia. Primary diseases of the bone marrow usually affect all hematopoietic cell lines. Anemia is a chronic change when the marrow is injured, because erythrocytes have a much longer half-life (120 days in the dog) than other blood cells. In most cases of nonregenerative anemia, the MCV and MCHC are within normal limits because there are few reticulocytes present. Therefore, the anemia can be described as a normocytic/normochromic anemia. The exceptions to this rule are FeLV-associated macrocytic nonregenerative anemia (macrocytic/normochromic) and chronic nonregenerative iron deficiency (microcytic and hypochromic).

Nonregenerative anemia due to secondary bone marrow disease is associated with renal disease (lack of erythropoietin), inflammatory disease (marrow suppressive inflammatory substances), and endocrine disease (lack of hormones that augment erythropoietin).

Polycythemia

Polycythemia is the counterpoint to anemia and is defined as an increase in red blood cell count, Hct/PCV, and hemoglobin. **The**

most common cause of polycythemia is dehydration. Dehydration-associated polycythemia is termed "relative" because the increase in red cell numbers is not due to increased production by the bone marrow. Instead, it is due to loss of the fluid portion of the blood due to dehydration. A high total protein will be present, in addition to the increased red cell parameters. All values will return to within their normal reference ranges with appropriate fluid therapy.

In contrast, absolute polycythemia is a real increase in red cell production. Absolute polycythemia can be a primary disease of the bone marrow, **polycythemia vera**, or due to inappropriate production of erythropoietin. Polycythemia vera is a neoplastic process that results in production of high numbers of red blood cells. Secondary, non–bone marrow causes of polycythemia are usually associated with diseases that cause general hypoxia (chronic pneumonia, large pulmonary or intrathoracic masses), renal hypoxia (masses that impinge on blood flow to the kidney), or neoplastic masses that produce excessive amounts of erythropoietin or erythropoietin-like substances (paraneoplastic syndromes). Table 4.7 lists causes of polycythemia. Clinical signs seen with increased numbers of red blood cells include injected (red) mucous membranes and distended blood vessels in the eye.

Leukocyte Changes Associated with Disease

Leukocyte changes in disease can affect each type of peripheral blood cell. Disease processes can decrease or increase the number of circulating leukocytes. The pattern of change in the absolute leukocyte numbers of each cell type is used to identify underlying diseases that are inflammatory (infectious and noninfectious), metabolic, and neoplastic, and to identify physiologic responses to excitement and stress. Understanding the mechanisms that cause changes in leukocyte number in response to both physiological stimuli and disease enables the veterinary technician to provide the most complete information to the clinician based on examination of the hemogram and peripheral blood film.

The total WBC count provides information on the total number of leukocytes and identifies a **leukocytosis** or a **leukopenia**. The differential cell count provides the absolute number of each leukocyte and allows a full characterization of the leukocytosis or leukopenia (i.e., a leukogram pattern). Each leukogram pattern can be used to develop a list of possible disease processes (a differential diagnosis). In addition to determining the absolute number of each type of leukocyte, examination of the leukocytes during the differential cell count identifies changes in leukocyte morphology that will provide valuable insight into possible disease processes. This section describes the mechanisms that affect the number of each leukocyte type and the morphological changes seen in specific leukocytes in response to either physiological changes or disease. Several atypical cell types are discussed.

Table 4.7. Types of polycythemia.

Relative	Dehydration, splenic contraction
Absolute primary	Polycythemia vera
Absolute secondary	Hypoxia (general)
	Renal hypoxia (renal masses)
	Erythropoietin-like substance produced by nonrenal neoplasia

Changes in Neutrophil Numbers and Morphology

Neutrophils

A thorough understanding of neutrophil dynamics, as discussed in Chapter 3, is essential to understanding alterations in neutrophil numbers due to physiological processes or disease. Inflammation, stress, and excitement each have a distinct effect on the neutrophil pools. As a short review, there are three neutrophil compartments: the proliferating pool, the maturation/storage pool, and the circulating/marginated pool. The proliferating and maturation/storage pools are in the bone marrow, and the circulating/marginated pool is in the blood vessels. Shifts of neutrophils among these pools are responsible for both increases in circulating neutrophils (**neutrophilia**) and decreases in circulating neutrophils (**neutropenia**).

Neutrophils in different stages of maturation are found in the different neutrophil pools. The proliferation pool contains neutrophil precursors that are still able to divide, (**myeloblasts, promyelocytes, and myelocytes**). The maturation/storage pool contains the remainder of the neutrophils in the bone marrow (**metamyelocytes, band neutrophils**, and **mature segmented neutrophils**). The storage subgroup in this pool consists of approximately a 5–7 day supply of mature neutrophils. When this storage pool of mature neutrophils is exhausted by an inflammatory demand for neutrophils, band neutrophils and, if demand is severe enough, metamyelocytes are released. When there is an overwhelming demand for neutrophils, myelocytes may be released from the proliferation pool. The circulating/marginated pool consists of mature neutrophils in the normal animal. The subgroup of neutrophils in this pool is marginated cells, neutrophils that line the blood vessel wall. The remaining neutrophils are in the circulating subgroup and are flowing within a central core of blood that is surrounded by cell-poor plasma. It is the circulating neutrophils in this core that are sampled when blood is drawn (Figure 4.12).

Neutrophilia

There are three primary mechanisms that can result in neutrophilia: inflammation, stress (increased circulating corticosteroids), and excitement (increased circulating epinephrine). Differentiating among these three causes can be difficult.

Inflammatory neutrophilia develops because of a demand for neutrophils in the tissues, in response to either tissue death (**necrosis**) or an infectious agent such as bacteria or fungi (**sepsis**). In most cases, a small focus of tissue inflammation will not cause a significant increase in circulating neutrophil numbers. However, a large lesion or an inflammatory process that affects multiple tissues (systemic inflammation) will result in an increase in the number of circulating neutrophils. If the inflammatory disease is severe or widespread enough, the demand for neutrophils will exhaust the maturation/storage pool of mature neutrophils and immature neutrophils will be released into the circulation.

The release of immature neutrophils is called a **left-shift**. The presence of a left-shift is diagnostic for an inflammatory leukogram. An inflammatory leukogram can be characterized by neutrophilia, normal neutrophil count, or neutropenia. The severity of the inflammatory process can be inferred by the severity of the left-shift. A left-shift is classified as regenerative or nonregenerative. Another way to refer to it is compensated or noncompensated. If the bone marrow can compensate fairly well for an inflammatory demand for neutrophils, the compensated inflammatory leukogram will show neutrophilia with a left-shift and the

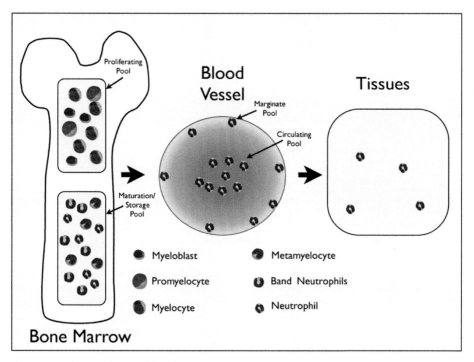

Figure 4.12. The normal neutrophil pools.

number of immature neutrophils will be less than the number of mature neutrophils.

If the bone marrow cannot adequately respond to the demand for neutrophils, three types of noncompensated inflammatory leukogram can be seen: one with neutrophilia in which the number of immature neutrophils outnumber the mature neutrophils, one in which there is a normal neutrophil count and there are increased numbers of immature neutrophils, and one in which there is a neutropenia and an increase in the number of immature neutrophils. It is important to remember that for the last two types of noncompensated inflammatory leukogram, the number of immature neutrophils does not have to exceed the number of mature neutrophils. Figure 4.13 illustrates three types of inflammatory leukogram and their classification.

Band neutrophils are considered the hallmark of an inflammatory leukogram. When band neutrophils are present in increased numbers, the clinician should be prompted to search for the focus of inflammation. It is very important that all technicians in the clinic who review blood films have a standard by which they identify a band neutrophil. The definition of a band neutrophil is a neutrophil whose nucleus is not segmented. Neutrophils in dogs and cats have less distinct segmentation than other species (i.e., humans and horses). In the dog and cat, a good rule of thumb is this: if the nucleus of the neutrophil does not have a narrow region that is less than 1/2 the greatest width of the remaining nucleus, it is a band neutrophil (Figure 4.14).

Once an inflammatory leukogram is identified, there are morphological changes in

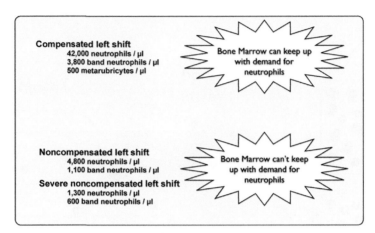

Compensated left shift
42,000 neutrophils / µl
3,800 band neutrophils / µl
500 metarubricytes / µl

Bone Marrow can keep up with demand for neutrophils

Noncompensated left shift
4,800 neutrophils / µl
1,100 band neutrophils / µl
Severe noncompensated left shift
1,300 neutrophils / µl
600 band neutrophils / µl

Bone Marrow can't keep up with demand for neutrophils

Figure 4.13. Types of left-shifts associated with inflammation.

the neutrophil that can assist in differentiating inflammation secondary to sepsis from inflammation secondary to nonseptic processes. Toxic neutrophils are most often seen with septic inflammatory processes. A toxic neutrophil has increased cytoplasmic basophilia and a "moth-eaten" or foamy change to its cytoplasm. In dogs, the presence of Dohlé bodies—angular, basophilic cytoplasmic inclusions—also indicate toxic change (Figure 4.15). Cat neutrophils often have Dohlé bodies without any change in cytoplasmic basophilia or vacuolation; therefore, these inclusions are not significant in the cat.

A compensated left-shift is seen with chronic or focal inflammation because neither process overwhelms the bone marrow

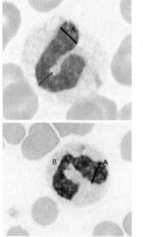

Band comparing the widest part of the nucleus (A) to the thinnest part of the nucleus (B): Line B is longer then 1/2 of line A

Neutrophil comparing the widest part of the nucleus (A) to the thinnest part of the nucleus (B): Line B is shorter then 1/2 of line A

Figure 4.14. A method for defining the band neutrophil.

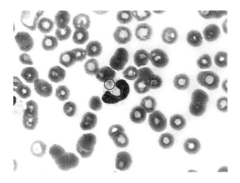

Figure 4.15. Dohlé body in a dog band neutrophil.

storage pool. The bone marrow can increase the rate of neutrophil production and keep up with the demand for the neutrophils in the inflamed tissue. Figure 4.16 illustrates the changes in the neutrophil pools in a compensated left-shift.

A decompensated left-shift occurs when inflammation has overwhelmed the bone marrow's ability to produce neutrophils in adequate number to meet the demands of the inflamed tissues. Overwhelming infections of whole organs such as pneumonia, pyelonephritis, open pyometra, generalized exudative dermatitis, and severe enteritis are often associated with a decompensated left-shift. Figure 4.17 illustrates the changes in the neutrophil pools with a decompensated left-shift.

Not all inflammatory leukograms have a left-shift or toxic change. Many animals with a mild or moderate inflammatory process will have a simple neutrophilia. As a result, it is often difficult to differentiate neutrophilia due to inflammation from neutrophilia due to stress (steroid-induced neutrophilia) or excitement (epinephrine-induced neutrophilia). There are hints in the

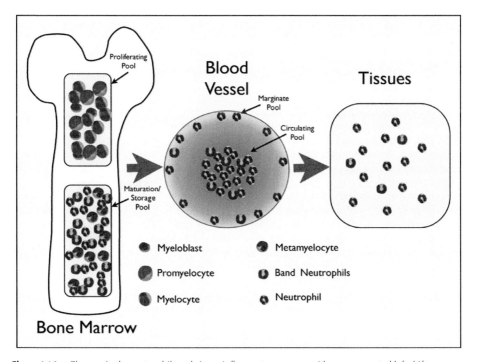

Figure 4.16. Changes in the neutrophil pools in an inflammatory process with a compensated left-shift.

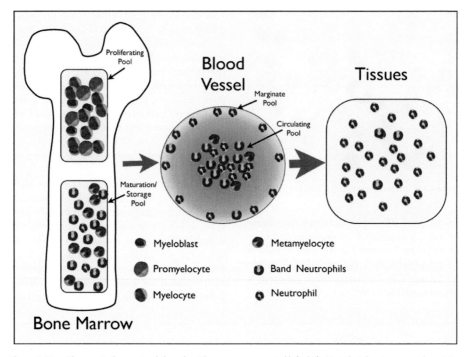

Figure 4.17. Changes in the neutrophil pools with a noncompensated left-shift. Note that the storage pool contains no mature neutrophils.

remainder of the leukogram that can help. A steroid or stress response is also associated with decreased numbers of lymphocytes, and in the dog, an increased number of monocytes. An excitement response is often associated with a concurrent increase in lymphocytes.

Neutrophilia associated with stress is caused by the effects of corticosteroids on the movement of neutrophils between the neutrophil pools. Steroids increase the release of neutrophils from the storage pool and increase retention of neutrophils in the circulation by making them less "sticky" (decreasing the number of neutrophils in the marginated pool) and less flexible. These changes prevent neutrophils from easily exiting the circulating into the tissues. Figure 4.18 illustrates the changes in the neutrophil pools due to the effects of increased circu-

lating steroids. The effect of steroids on neutrophils is one of the reasons patients that are receiving steroids are more susceptible to infections; their neutrophils cannot exit into the tissues to destroy bacteria during an infection. An excellent example of this is the development of bacterial cystitis in patients with increased circulating corticosteroids due to either a disease or administration of large doses of steroid medication. In these individuals, the urine does not always have a significant number of neutrophils in response to the bacteria present.

Increased circulating epinephrine in the excited patient will cause an increase in blood pressure that "washes" marginated neutrophils off of the vessel wall into the circulating pool resulting in apparent neutrophilia. A **lymphocytosis** is also seen in conjunction with neutrophilia and can at

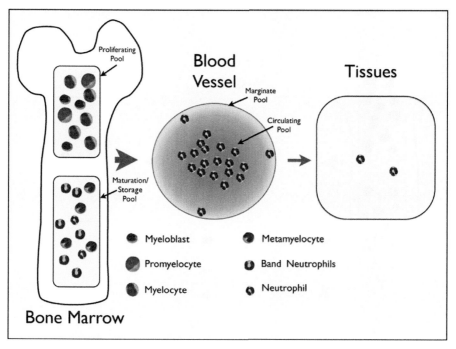

Figure 4.18. Changes in the neutrophil pools due to increased circulating steroids (stress neutrophilia). Note that there is increased release of mature neutrophils from the storage pool and decreased numbers of neutrophils in the marginated pool causing a neutrophilia. Because the neutrophils cannot attach to the wall of the vessel they cannot migrate into the tissues.

times exceed the number of neutrophils. This response is more prominent in the cat because cats have a larger marginated pool compared to the dog. Figure 4.19 illustrates the changes in the circulating neutrophil pool in response to excitement.

Neutropenia

Inflammatory leukograms can also be seen with decreased neutrophil numbers (**neutropenia**). Severe inflammation can so greatly overwhelm the bone marrow that it cannot maintain neutrophil numbers at the normal level. In this case, a left-shift and toxic change are usually present. Neutropenia does not always indicate inflammation. Bone marrow injury can cause de-

creased production of neutrophils, often in association with a nonregenerative anemia and thrombocytopenia. Infectious agents (panleukopenia virus, chronic ehrlichiosis) and drugs (chemotherapeutic drugs, estrogen, certain antibiotics) can cause reversible damage to the bone marrow. In these cases, treatment of the infection or withdrawal of the drug will allow the remnant hematopoietic stem cells to repopulate the marrow. Irreversible damage to the marrow is often seen with prolonged exposure to certain drugs, replacement of the marrow hematopoietic tissue by a neoplastic process, or as an idiopathic process. In these cases, aggressive treatment to stimulate the bone marrow fails because there are no hematopoietic stem cells left to repopulate the bone marrow.

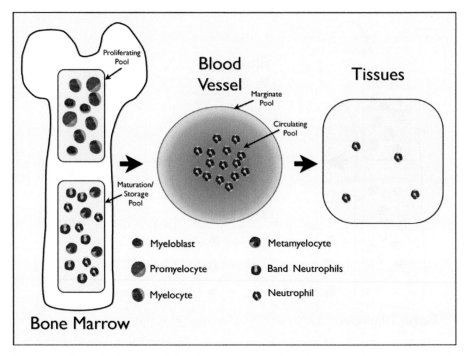

Figure 4.19. Changes in the neutrophil pools due to increased circulating epinephrine (excitement). The marginated pool is the only pool affected by excitement.

One special case of neutropenia is due to gram-negative bacterial sepsis. Gram-negative bacteria such as *Escherichia coli* and *Klebsiella* spp. have a component of their cell wall called endotoxin or lipopolysaccharide (LPS). Endotoxin has many potent effects that contribute to the serious clinical signs seen in patients with gram-negative bacterial infections. One of these effects is to increase the "stickiness" of neutrophils, prompting neutrophils in the circulating core to enter the marginated pool. Endotoxin also inhibits the release of neutrophils from the maturation/storage pool and decreases the rate of proliferation and maturation of neutrophils. Each of these effects contributes to the development of neutropenia. Figure 4.20 illustrates the changes in the neutrophil pools in response to endotoxin. The effects of endotoxin can

be seen within 15 minutes of exposure to the toxin. Just as rapidly as the neutrophil count can drop, the neutrophil count can rebound with remarkable neutrophilia with a left-shift when the animal is successfully treated.

Changes in Lymphocyte Numbers in Disease

Lymphocytosis

Lymphocytosis is an increase in the number of circulating lymphocytes. As discussed previously, excitement can cause a significant lymphocytosis and is likely the most common cause of this leukogram change.

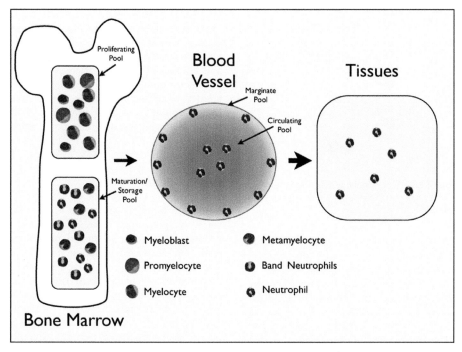

Figure 4.20. Changes in the neutrophil pools in sepsis (endotoxin). Note that there is a decrease in the number of neutrophils released by the storage pool and an increase in the number of neutrophils in the marginated pool. This results in a decreased number of neutrophils in the circulating pool (neutropenia).

Vaccination in young dogs and cats is also associated with a significant increase in circulating lymphocytes as a result of strong antigenic stimulation of the immune system. The increase in lymphocytes is seen 1 to 2 weeks after vaccination. The lymphocytes seen in this case, as with excitement, are small and normal in appearance. Occasionally, large lymphocytes with deeply basophilic cytoplasm and prominent nucleoli (**immunoblasts**) can be seen as a component of the lymphocytosis (Figure 4.21).

Both excitement-induced lymphocytosis and lymphocytosis secondary to vaccination are considered physiological lymphocytosis. A less common, but important, cause of lymphocytosis is lymphoid leukemia. There are two types of lymphoid leukemia, acute or lymphoblastic and

chronic or lymphocytic. The lymphocytes seen in lymphoblastic leukemia are large and have prominent nucleoli and variably

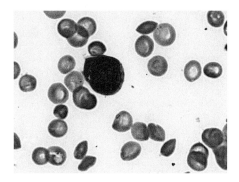

Figure 4.21. A large reactive lymphocyte in a puppy postvaccination.

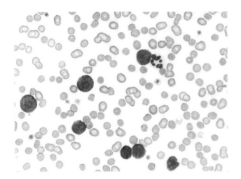

Figure 4.22. Acute lymphoid leukemia. Note the size of the lymphoid cells compared to the one neutrophil in the field.

basophilic cytoplasm (Figure 4.22). This neoplastic process is easily distinguished from a physiological lymphocytosis.

On the other hand, chronic or lymphocytic leukemia can be difficult to differentiate from physiological lymphocytosis because, in both cases, the circulating lymphocytes are small and have normal morphology (Figure 4.23). The clinician will have to use other factors to decide whether a dog or cat with a lymphocytic lymphocytosis has a neoplastic or physiological process.

There is one special case of lymphocytosis that is associated with an infectious disease: ehrlichiosis. Rickettsial organisms, the cause of ehrlichiosis, are parasites of

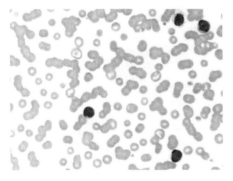

Figure 4.23. Chronic lymphocytic leukemia. Note the normal morphology of the small lymphocytes.

neutrophils, monocytes, and platelets. The monocytic parasite (*Ehrlichia canis*) can cause a marked lymphocytosis where the lymphocytes are slightly larger than normal and have small numbers of eosinophilic to slightly basophilic granules, often nestled in a small niche in the nucleus. The distinctive morphology of these granulated lymphocytes should prompt testing for ehrlichiosis.

Lymphopenia

Decreased numbers of circulating lymphocytes, lymphopenia, is seen with several processes. Stress, as discussed previously, results in decreased lymphocytes because steroids inhibit the return of lymphocytes to the circulation and can cause lysis of lymphocytes (**lympholysis**). Lymphopenia can be due to loss of lymphocytes into the tissues and body cavities. **Chylothorax** is an accumulation of lymphocyte-rich fluid (lymph) in the thoracic cavity. Lymphocytes can also be lost or compartmentalized (sequestered) in dilated lymphatic vessels of the gastrointestinal tract (**lymphangiectasia**). Hereditary immune-deficiency diseases can result in the decreased production of lymphocytes, and viral disease can result in the necrosis of lymphoid tissues and destruction of lymphocytes.

Monocytes

Monocytosis, increased circulating monocytes, is a feature of the stress leukogram in the dog. Tissue necrosis and some forms of chronic inflammation, such as fungal disease, are also associated with monocytosis as a component of the inflammatory leukogram. Occasionally, monocytosis is seen in neutropenia patients, perhaps as a compensation for the lack of neutrophils. A decreased number of monocytes is not associated with disease.

Eosinophils

Eosinophilia, increased numbers of circulating eosinophils, is most commonly associated with diseases of hypersensitivity or allergy (allergic dermatitis, asthma), parasitism (heartworm disease and some external parasites), eosinophilic enteritis, and hypereosinophilic syndrome. Although eosinophils are routinely seen in the tissues of animals with fungal disease and mast cell tumor, these diseases are not commonly associated with an eosinophilia. Increased numbers of basophils, basophilia, can be seen in concert with eosinophilia. Basophilia is rarely seen by itself.

Atypical Circulating Leukocytes

Atypical circulating leukocytes are often indications of neoplasia or leukemia. If routine evaluation of a peripheral blood film reveals atypical cells in addition to the normal peripheral blood leukocytes, it is best to have the blood film and a fresh blood sample sent into a reference laboratory for a pathology review. Determining the origin of neoplastic cells in peripheral blood may require specialized testing in addition to review of the Wright-Giemsa stained slide. Figure 4.24 illustrates several examples of neoplastic leukocytes.

There are hereditary disorders that are characterized by circulating abnormal leukocytes. Pelger-Huët anomaly is a genetic disease found in many breeds of dog and occasional cats. In individuals affected with Pelger-Huët anomaly, all circulating neutrophils and eosinophils are hyposegmented and resemble band forms of these granulocytes. There is no disease process associated with this anomaly. It can cause significant confusion when a perfectly healthy-appearing dog has what would be a noncompensated left-shift in any other patient. One of the keys to identifying a patient with Pelger-Huët anomaly is the fact that the eosinophils are affected as well as the neutrophils and that the neutrophils have dense clumped nuclear chromatin and no evidence of toxic change

Chediak-Higashi syndrome, mucopolysaccharidosis VI, and **gangliosidosis** are all rare inherited diseases that have abnormal leukocytes. The neutrophils from individuals with Chediak-Higashi have a small number of lightly eosinophilic, moderately sized granules. The neutrophils from individuals with mucopolysaccharidosis VI have numerous small basophilic granules, and occasionally their lymphocytes have vacuoles. Individuals with gangliosidosis have vacuolated lymphocytes. Figure 4.25 illustrates the leukocyte morphology of these inherited diseases.

Infectious Disease Agents of Erythrocytes and Leukocytes

There are several infectious diseases that can directly affect the hemogram findings. Most erythroparasites are associated with anemia. The severity of the anemia depends on the individual infectious agent and, in some cases, the age of the patient.

Mycoplasma hemofelis and *Mycoplasma hemominutum* are two erythroparasites that attach to the surface of the erythrocyte. They are small and can be difficult to identify unless the blood film is well stained and free of stain precipitate. *Mycoplasma hemominutum* is the smaller of the two organisms and is usually seen as a small, rod-shaped, dark-staining body on the edge of the erythrocyte. *Mycoplasma hemofelis* is larger and may form distinct signet ring forms that can be seen overlying the erythrocyte on the blood film. In many cases, only one of these organisms will be seen on the blood film. Some cats can be infected by both. *Mycoplasma hemofelis* is the organism that is most often associated with

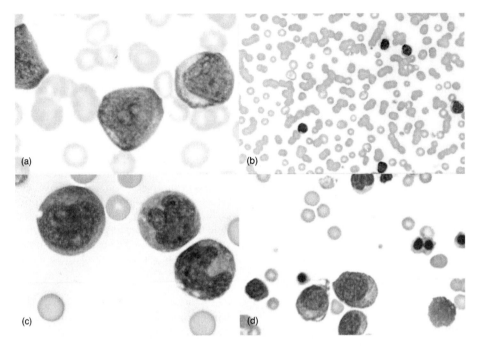

Figure 4.24. **(a)** Acute lymphoid leukemia. **(b)** Chronic lymphocytic leukemia. **(c)** Myelomonocytic leukemia. **(d)** Erythremic myelosis (erythroleukemia).

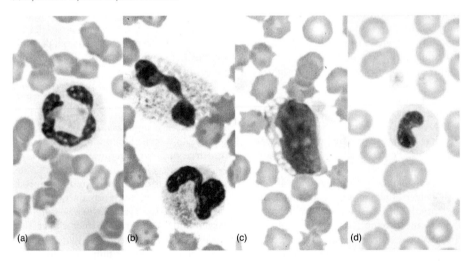

Figure 4.25. **(a)** Neutrophils with two eosinophilic granules from a cat with Chediak-Higashi syndrome. **(b)** Neutrophils with numerous basophilic granules from a cat with mucopolysaccharidosis. **(c)** Lymphocyte with numerous discrete vacuoles from a cat with GM1-gangliocytosis. **(d)** Neutrophil from a dog with Pelger-Huët anomaly.

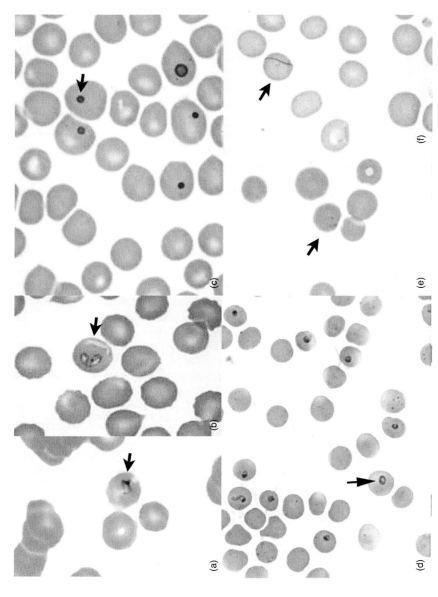

Figure 4.26. (a) *Babesia gibsoni.* (b) *Babesia canis.* (c) Canine distemper virus inclusions. (d) *Cytauxzoan felis.* (e) *Mycoplasma hemofelis.* (f) *Mycoplasma hemocanis.*

anemia (extravascular hemolytic anemia). *Mycoplasma hemominutum* can be seen in nonanemic cats. The feline mycoplasma organisms are spread by bites and blood sucking external parasites such as fleas. *Mycoplasma hemocanis* is seen in dogs that are splenectomized or have poor splenic function. It is rarely, if ever, seen in dogs with a functional spleen.

Babesia canis and *Babesia gibsoni* are internal erythroparasites that are within the erythrocyte cytoplasm. Though rare in the United State, **babesiosis** is still seen on occasion. Babesia organisms are protozoa rather than bacteria. The disease is spread by ticks and bites. *Babesia canis* is the larger of the two organisms. It is usually shaped like a teardrop and may be found as a pair within one erythrocyte. *Babesia gibsoni* is significantly smaller than *Babesia canis* and has a signet ring shape with a small dark nucleus at the periphery of a clear vacuole-like space. The American bulldog and the pit bull appear to have an increased susceptibility to *Babesia gibsoni*.

Cytauxzoon felis is a protozoan erythroparasite of cats similar in appearance to *Babesia gibsoni*. They are small signet ring structures with a small dark nucleus and a clear vacuolar space within the cytoplasm of the erythrocyte. When first reported, cytauxzoonosis was an invariably fatal disease in cats. In most cases, by the time the owner noted that the cat was ill and presented their pet to the hospital, the patient was moribund and died shortly after arrival. Over time, the parasite appears to have developed a better relationship with its new host, the domestic cat. More cats are surviving treatment in recent years. This parasite is most commonly seen in the central and southern states.

Canine distemper virus, though rarely identified on routine blood film examination, can be seen in dogs with very acute disease. Fortunately, as a result of excellent vaccination programs, most practices in the United State see only rare cases of this

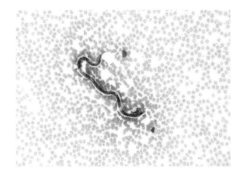

Figure 4.27. Microfiliaria in a blood film from a dog positive for *Dirofilaria immitis* antigen.

devastating viral disease of young dogs. In acute infections, viral inclusion can be seen in neutrophils and erythrocytes. The inclusions are best seen using Diff-Quik stain and appear as deep magenta homogeneous inclusions. They are easily missed on Wright-Giemsa stain because they stain light lavender and fade into the background staining of the neutrophil and erythrocyte cytoplasm. Figure 4.26 illustrates the morphology of several infectious agents that can be seen on a peripheral blood film.

Dirofilaria immitis (the canine heartworm) is a filarial worm seen primarily in dogs (occasionally in cats). The adults live in the anterior vena cava, right atrium, and occasionally the right ventricle of the heart. The larvae (microfilaria) produced by the adult female worms can be seen in the peripheral blood in infected animals. The larvae are elongate and contain numerous small nuclei throughout their length. When microfilaria are identified on a blood film, it is important to perform a heartworm antigen test to confirm that the microfilaria are *Dirofilaria immitis*. There are other less-pathogenic filarial worms that can release microfilaria into the blood (*Dipetalonema reconditum*). The larvae of these two species of filarial worms cannot be distinguished from each other on a blood film. Figure 4.27 illustrates a circulating microfilaria from a dog with confirmed heartworm disease.

Renal Physiology and Anatomy, Clinical Diagnostics, and Disease

Introduction

Before discussing renal function and its clinical diagnostics, sample handling technique must be reviewed. In handling blood in a serum separator or clot tube (red top tube), team members must evaluate the tube for changes suggestive of artifact or pathology. Just as the purple top tube can help detect changes in the blood that can suggest artifact (i.e., clotting) or disease (i.e., agglutination), changes in the red top tube can also suggest disease or artifact that can affect the outcome of the clinical diagnostics.

Step 1

After blood is drawn from the patient, it should be placed in the red top tube by removing the red stopper and gently dripped into the tube itself. This prevents trauma to the red cells and helps to reduce artificial hemolysis. If the medical team member is using a vacutainer, the normal flow of blood into the tube by the vacuum pressure should not be strong enough to produce hemolysis.

Step 2

Allow the blood tube to clot. In general, 10–15 minutes should produce sufficient time to allow for the blood to clot in the red top tube. If a clot does not occur, it may suggest two possibilities: artifact or pathology.

Artifact

The blood has been contaminated with some EDTA while placing the blood in another tube (purple, blue, or green top). This can occur when using either a syringe or vacutainer system; a small amount of EDTA can contaminate the vacutainer delivery needle as blood is being transferred into the tube. This EDTA then can affect the blood entering the red or serum top tubes stopping the clotting process. To help prevent this artifact from occurring, team members using a vacutainer system should place blood into red top tube initially and then fill the other nonclotting tubes.

Pathology

If the patient is suffering from a disease that decreases platelets or clotting factors (see Chapter 13), the patient's ability to clot may be compromised. **Although it is important to note that with clotting or lack of clotting within the red top tube, the lack of a clot does not always reflect the patient's ability to clot in its body. A lack of clot in the red top tube should always be discussed with the veterinarian.** If a clot does not occur, the following samples could be collected to determine the patient's ability to clot blood:

Redraw a Venous Sample

Drawing another blood sample and placing the blood into another fresh red top tube will rule out the possibility that the previous sample was contaminated with EDTA. When drawing a fresh blood sample in this situation, **a jugular blood draw should not be attempted.** If the patient does have a clotting problem, a jugular draw can produce a very large collection of blood under the skin (**hematoma**) that can decrease the patient's red blood cell count to the level that a transfusion may be necessary.

Obtain a Clotting Time

Obtaining a clotting time from a peripheral vein can help the medical team evaluate the levels of chemical in the blood to help initiate the clotting process (**clotting factors;** (see Chapter 13)). Increased clotting times represent a life-threatening concern for the patient, which, when identified, should be discussed with the veterinarian immediately.

Evaluate the Platelet Count

Although it takes both clotting factors and platelets to produce a final clot formation, often patients that have increased clotting times will also have decreased platelet numbers. The platelets are consumed as the body tries to initiate the clotting cascade and stop internal bleeding. As with clotting factors, a patient with decreased platelet counts (<60,000) can represent a life-threatening concern for the patient, which, when identified, should be discussed with the veterinarian immediately.

Step 3

Evaluate the serum for abnormality. Once a clot is observed, the sample should be spun down in the centrifuge for 15 minutes. Once the blood tube is removed from the centrifuge, the serum should be evaluated for abnormality. Normal serum is a clear straw color. Changes to the serum can occur due to artifact or disease; these changes not only can suggest disease but can also artifactually affect other components of the blood chemistry. **Any changes in the blood serum should be documented in the chart immediately and discussed with the veterinarian.** The following abnormalities can be noted in the serum.

White Serum (Lipemia)

Lipemia suggests an increased white precipitate of fat or lipid in the serum. This can occur artifactually if the animal has eaten a fatty meal before the blood draw. This also this seems to be a common artifact noted when drawing blood from miniature schnauzers. Any disease that alters the body's ability to digest and metabolize fat can also cause a true lipemia. Diseases that produce a true lipemia are diabetes mellitus, hypothyroidism, hyperadrenocorticism, hyperlipidemia (rare), and hypercholesterolemia (rare). Dependent on the chemistry unit used, lipemia can also artifactually alter liver and other blood chemistries.

Red Serum (Hemolysis)

Hemolysis occurs when red blood cells are destroyed releasing hemoglobin into the serum. This can occur artifactually due to a traumatic blood draw or improper transfer of blood into the red top tube. In disease conditions, hemolysis can be noted in the early stages of **immune-mediated hemolytic anemia (IMHA)**, where the red blood cells are being attacked by white blood cells like foreign bacteria. Dependent on the chemistry unit used, hemolysis can also artifactually alter liver (especially bilirubin), kidney, blood calcium, and other blood chemistries.

Yellow Serum (Jaundice)

There is no artifact that can produce jaundice. Jaundice occurs when **bilirubin,** a waste product from red blood cell production, builds up in the tissue. Bilirubin normally is produced by the body as red blood cells are destroyed in the spleen and then converted into a nontoxic form in the liver. It is then excreted by the liver through the gallbladder. Animals develop jaundice with liver disease, gallbladder obstruction, or massive destruction of red blood cells in the blood vessels (secondary to IMHA).

Urogenital System

The urogenital system consists of the kidneys, ureters, bladder, urethra, and reproductive organs of the animal. The kidneys are a complicated organ responsible for filtering toxin out of blood, concentrating urine to prevent dehydration, controlling blood electrolyte levels, controlling blood pH (blood gas), and maintaining blood pressure.

Renal disease is one of the most common forms of geriatric disease in both the cat and dog. Team members must understand renal function, obtain a thorough database to help identify renal disease, understand blood chemistry changes that identify renal disease, and be able to discuss these concerns with the client.

The urinary system's main function is to control the elimination of waste and toxins from the body. Severe disease occurs when the kidneys are unable to filter out toxins and waste through specialized structures called **glomeruli (Bowman's capsules)** (renal cortex) and concentrate the urine by reabsorbing water in the **loops of Henle** (renal medulla) to prevent the fluid loss that produces dehydration. Further, the kidneys also function to help produce red blood cells from the bone marrow, control blood pressure through a cellular mechanism called the **renin-angiotensin system,** control the excretion of acidifying compounds that help to control blood pH, and balance of the electrolytes (sodium and potassium) within the body. Normal kidney function is necessary for life.

Each animal has two kidneys, the right and the left (Figure 5.1). The kidneys are located close to the spine in the middle of the abdomen. The left kidney is slightly further behind the right kidney, which is located just behind the last rib. The right kidney is positioned within the rib cage. The right and left adrenal glands sit just in front of both kidneys. The internal anatomy of the kidneys is split into several sections, each section having its own anatomy and function.

The kidney's internal anatomy has two major anatomical regions, each of which has its own architecture and function. The **renal cortex** is responsible for the filtration of toxins out of the blood, balancing

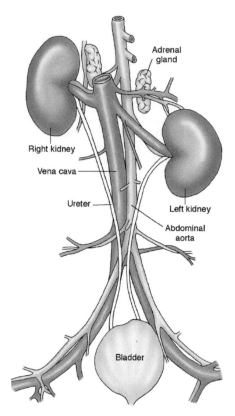

Figure 5.1. Illustration of renal position and local anatomy within the abdomen.

of blood electrolytes, and control of blood pressure. The **renal medulla** is responsible for the concentration of urine to prevent dehydration.

The renal cortex is the outermost region of kidney tissue. This region houses hundreds of thousands of glomeruli (Figure 5.2).

The glomeruli are closely associated with small arteriole beds. The glomerular filters have very fine openings (called fenestrations) that allow small molecules to filter into the tubules from the bloodstream. As blood passes through the small arteriole beds, all blood molecules small enough flow passively into the urinary

space. These smaller molecules are sugar, amino acids, waste products, and electrolytes (e.g., sodium, potassium, chloride, etc.). Larger blood molecules such as proteins (e.g., albumin, globulin, etc.) cannot pass through the small fenestrations of the healthy glomerular capsule.

Once the molecules and fluid have been passed into the urinary space, the urine flows on into the **proximal convoluted tubules**. The function of these tubules is to aggressively reabsorb all of the necessary nutrients back into the bloodstream. This is an active process accomplished by cellular pumps within the walls of the proximal and distal tubules. Once the necessary nutrients are reabsorbed, the fluid then passes into the loops of Henle within the renal medulla.

The loops of Henle function to reabsorb a large percentage of the fluid component of the urine (Figure 5.3).

To do this the cells of the nephrotic loops actively extract sodium ions (Na^+) and move them into the medullary tissue around the nephrotic loops. The tissue in this region is more concentrated than the fluid moving through the loops of Henle, causing water to passively move into the surrounding tissue. This process reabsorbs 2/3 of the fluid within the nephrotic loops. Initially, patients unable to actively reabsorb fluid from the urine first develop increased thirst (**polydipsia**) and urination (**polyuria**) as they try to compensate for increased fluid losses. As the disease progresses, animals experience life-threatening dehydration and are unable to make up their fluid losses.

Once the urine leaves the loops of Henle, it enters the collecting ducts and enters the renal pelvis. The renal pelvis collects all the urine produced before moving into the ureters. The ureters enter the bladder at the bladder's neck in the area called the **trigone**. Once urine collects in the bladder, it is excreted through urethra and leaves the body through the urethral opening.

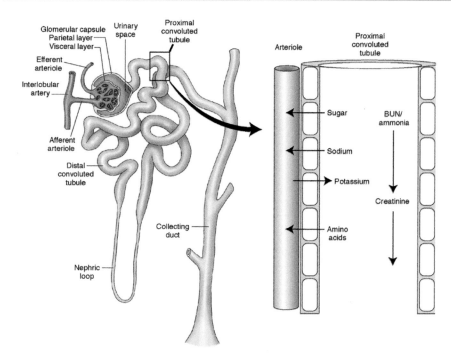

Figure 5.2. Illustration of a glomerular capsule, urinary space, proximal and distal convoluted tubules, nephrotic loops, and collecting ducts.

The kidneys must filter the blood at a constant rate in order to maintain a low level of blood toxins. To do this, 20% of the body's blood volume must be filtered through the kidneys every minute (Figure 5.4). Any disease or pathology that decreases **glomerular filtration** increases the amount of toxin in the form of ammonia in the bloodstream. This is called **azotemia.** The increase in toxins makes the patient weak, anorexic, and nauseous; causes diarrhea and vomiting; and can produce life-threatening dehydration and potential shock.

Evaluating Renal Function

Key elements in the chemistry allow the medical team to evaluate if normal renal filtration (**glomerular filtration;** Table 5.1) and urinary concentration **is occurring.**

Diseases, which effect the renal glomerular filtration, inhibit the kidney's ability to filter out toxins from the bloodstream. The inability of glomerular filtration is directly proportional to the amount of toxins within the bloodstream. In general, it takes 65–70% of all glomeruli to be affected before there is a rise in the renal toxins (azotemia) of **blood urea nitrogen (BUN)** and **creatinine.** The following sections describe blood chemistry parameters that can suggest decreased ability of glomerular filtration.

Blood Urea Nitrogen (BUN)

Blood urea nitrogen is an amalgamation of two ammonia molecules. Ammonia is

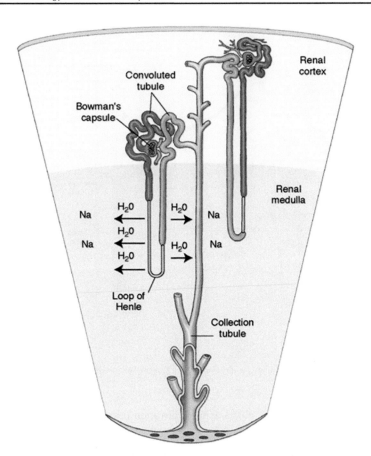

Figure 5.3. Illustration of a renal cortex and medulla. The renal medulla maintains a very high salt concentration that serves to pull fluid out of the urine. The concentrating ability of the kidneys helps to prevent dehydration of the patient.

a toxin produced during normal protein metabolism. BUN is produced in the liver and then placed into the bloodstream so that it can be excreted during normal glomerular filtration. General increases in BUN concentration can be associated with decreased glomerular filtration. However, intestinal bleeding can also increase BUN. Blood contains a large amount of protein, which, when bled into the intestinal system, is digested like any other food source. Diseases that produce intestinal bleeding (e.g., parvoviral infection) can secondarily increase BUN levels in the blood. Further, high protein meals can also produce a transient increase in serum BUN as the protein is metabolized. Although blood levels of BUN can vary from lab to lab, normal BUN levels are generally as shown in Chart 5.1.

Chart 5.1

Canine	10–26 mg/dL
Feline	15–34 mg/dL

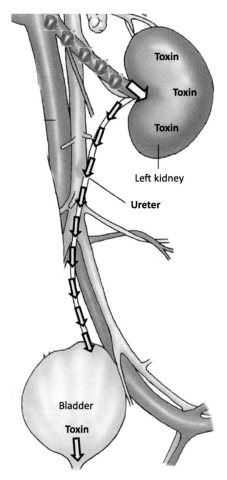

Figure 5.4. Image of normal filtration of blood. It requires 20% of blood volume going through the kidneys/minute to allow adequate removal of toxins from the blood into the urine.

creatinine. Although blood levels of creatinine can vary from lab to lab, normal creatinine levels are generally as shown in Chart 5.2.

Chart 5.2

Canine	0.5–1.3 mg/dL
Feline	1.0–2.2 mg/dL

Phosphorus

Phosphorus is a mineral that is a key element in many cell functions, including bone formation, energy metabolism, muscle contraction, and acid-base balance. Phosphorus is largely excreted by the kidneys. There are many causes for increased blood phosphorus levels (**hyperphosphotemia**, see Chapter 8); however, the presence of hyperphosphotemia in association with elevations of BUN and creatinine can support changes in glomerular filtration. Although blood levels of phosphorus can vary from lab to lab, normal phosphorus levels are generally as shown in Chart 5.3.

Chart 5.3

Canine	2.3–5.5 mg/dL
Feline	3.0–7.0 mg/dL

Creatinine

Creatinine is an amino acid that is a metabolite of muscle, which is produced in the body during normal muscle metabolism. Increases in creatinine concentration is directly associated with a decrease in glomerular filtration. Unlike BUN, there are no secondary causes for elevations in

Albumin

Albumin is protein produced in the liver and released in the bloodstream to carry molecules throughout the body. If glomerular filters are damaged, albumin can pass from the blood into the urine during normal glomerular filtration (Figure 5.5).

Protein loss into the urine can occur early in renal disease before a true azotemia

Table 5.1.   Clinical diagnostics that help to monitor kidney function.

Element	Chemistry Elements That Suggest Decreased Glomerular Filtration	Other Factors That Elevate Enzyme or Element Level Besides Decrease in Glomerular Filtration	Factors Indicating That True Renal Azotemia
BUN	Azotemia BUN >26 mg/dL (Canine) BUN >34 mg/dL (Feline)	GI bleeding High protein meal	USG <1.015
Creatinine	Azotemia Crea >1.3 mg/dL (Canine) Crea >2.2 mg/dL (Feline)	None	USG <1.015
Phosphorus	P >5.5 mg/dL (Canine) P >7.0 mg/dL (Feline)	Disease that affects calcium and phosphorus balance.	Increased phosphorus must be in association with elevated BUN/creatinine and low USG.
Potassium	K <4.0 mEq/L (Canine) K <3.7 mEq/L (Feline)	Any disease that can cause fluid losses (i.e., vomiting, anorexia, or diarrhea may lower body potassium)	Decreased potassium must be in association with elevated BUN/creatinine and low USG.
Potassium	K >5.4 mEq/L (Canine) K >5.2 mEq/L (Feline)	Hypoadrenocorticism (Addison's Dz)	Increased potassium must be in association with elevated BUN/creatinine and urinary obstruction. CAN BE ACUTELY LIFE THREATENING
Albumin	Alb <3.1 g/dL (Canine) Alb <2.4 g/dL (Feline)	Liver Disease Bleeding Gastrointestinal Dz	Possible early warning of impending renal disease. Low albumin must be associated with a true renal proteinuria (See Chapter 11)

is noted. A combination of low body al-bumin (**hypoalbuminemia**) and high uri-nary protein levels (**proteinuria**) can suggest glomerular damage and be an early indica-tor of renal disease. Although blood levels of albumin can vary from lab to lab, nor-mal albumin levels are generally as shown in Chart 5.4.

Chart 5.4

Canine	3.1–4.5 g/dL
Feline	2.4–4.1 g/dL

Potassium

Potassium is an intracellular ion that helps produce electrical energy allowing skeletal and cardiac contraction muscle, depolariza-tion of nerves, and other metabolic func-tions (see Chapter 8). Potassium is normally absorbed through the digestive system, stored inside cells, and excreted through the kidneys. Although many diseases can alter blood potassium levels, chronic re-nal disease can produce a profoundly low body potassium level (**hypokalemia**). This

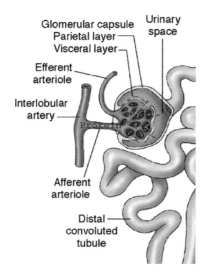

Glomerular capsule
Parietal layer
Visceral layer
Urinary space
Efferent arteriole
Interlobular artery
Afferent arteriole
Distal convoluted tubule

Figure 5.5. Illustration of kidneys with damage to the filters causing blood protein (albumin) to pass into the urinary space.

occurs as the patient loses its ability to concentrate urine, and more and more potassium is excreted from the body with larger quantities of urine. Although blood levels of potassium can vary from lab to lab, normal potassium levels are generally as shown in Chart 5.5.

Chart 5.5

| Canine | 4.0–5.4 mEq/L |
| Feline | 3.7–5.2 mEq/L |

Diseases that alter renal medullary tissue affect the animal's ability to concentrate urine. These animals have lost the ability of reabsorbing sodium into the medullary tissue and are unable to create a high sodium gradient. This stops the flow of water out of the urine and into the tissue, increasing fluid loss. Patients with decreased medullary function cannot maintain normal hydration. To help compensate for the loss, patients begin to drink large amounts of water. Often these pets will begin to show in-

creased thirst and urination as a first symptom to these diseases.

The kidney's ability to concentrate urine is measured by an instrument called a **refractometer** (see Chapter 9). This instrument measures the concentration of a fluid. The specific gravity of fluids is measured from 1.001 to above 1.045. The higher the number, the more concentrated the fluid. A urine specific gravity is the best assessment of concentrating ability of the renal medulla and a key indicator of renal disease.

To diagnose true renal disease the medical team must prove that the patient has lost the ability to both filter toxins (azotemia) and concentrate urine. If both elements are not observable, the patient may be affected by a secondary disease that affects either glomerular filtration or medullary concentration. It then becomes the medical team's responsibility to differentiate primary kidney disease vs. another disease affecting renal function (Algorithm 5.1).

Prerenal azotemia is caused by decreased blood perfusion of the kidneys, producing decreased glomerular filtration. This syndrome is not caused by kidney disease but is caused by **dehydration**. Elevated percentage of dehydration decreases the body's ability to perfuse its organs normally, and glomerular filtration decreases. However, the kidneys still maintain the ability to concentrate urine (Figure 5.6).

Text Box 5.1

Key Points to Help Distinguish Prerenal Azotemia

- The pet has evidence of decreased glomerular filtration with an increased azotemia.
- Urine specific gravity is high because the kidneys have not lost their ability to concentrate urine.
- The azotemia reverts to normal levels after hydration is restored.

Algorithm 5.1. Overview of diagnosis of renal disease

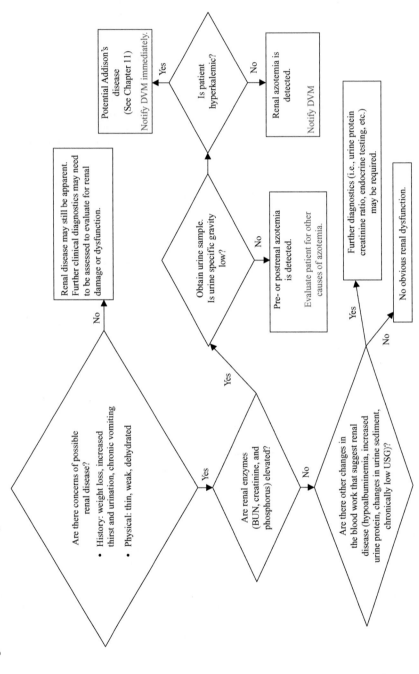

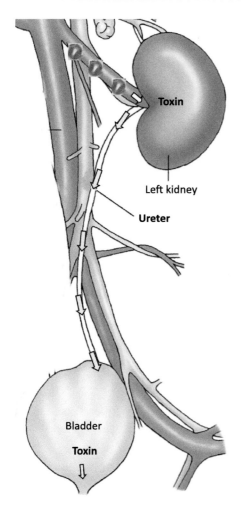

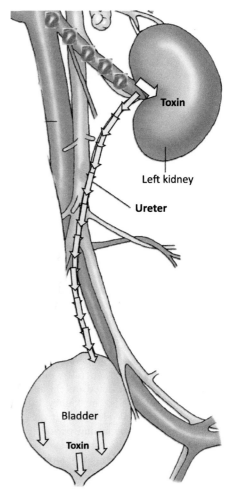

Figure 5.6. Illustration of prerenal azotemia. Dehydration decreases blood flow through the kidneys slowing glomerular filtration and reduces the amount of toxins in the urine. This causes increasing levels of toxins in the bloodstream.

Figure 5.7. Due to the loss of 2/3–3/4 of kidney mass, the kidneys cannot adequately filter or concentrate urine. This produces patients with severe azotemia (high levels of toxins in the blood/low levels of toxins in the urine) and patients that produce large amounts of urine because the kidneys have lost the ability to concentrate urine.

In **renal azotemia,** a disease that primarily affects the kidneys causes azotemia and decreased medullary concentration. In order for the azotemia to occur, 65–75% damage to both kidneys must occur. The kidneys have lost the ability to concentrate urine; therefore, the urine specific gravity can be much lower than normal (<1.015). With severe chronic renal disease, the azotemia may not revert to normal with fluid therapy (Figure 5.7).

Text Box 5.2

Key Points with Renal Azotemia

- The pet has evidence of decreased glomerular filtration with an increased azotemia.
- Urine specific gravity is low because the kidneys have lost their ability to concentrate urine.
- The azotemia does not generally revert to normal levels after hydration is restored.

In **postrenal azotemia**, there is a rise in kidney nonprotein nitrogenous compounds due to an obstruction of the bladder, which produces a retrograde backflow of urine to the kidneys and ammonia into the bloodstream (Figure 5.8). A severe azotemia is present; however, urine specific gravity tends to be high initially because the kidneys still maintain the ability to concentrate urine. Due to lack of potassium excretion, a life-threatening high blood potassium level (**hyperkalemia**, see Chapter 8) can occur. Generally, once the urinary tract is unobstructed and the animal is rehydrated on fluids, the kidney values can return to normal. However, if the patient is obstructed for a long period (e.g., hours), the increased retrograde urinary pressure can produce permanent kidney disease. These patients come in obstructed and have life-threatening azotemia and dilute urine.

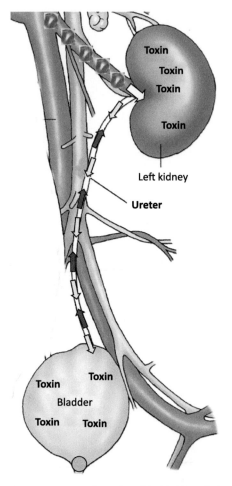

Figure 5.8. Due to obstruction of the bladder and urinary outflow tract, toxins that are pushed into the urine retrograde back into the kidneys, slowing glomerular filtration and producing severe azotemia. If obstructed long enough, permanent kidney disease can occur.

Text Box 5.3

Key Points with Postrenal Azotemia:

- The pet has evidence of decreased glomerular filtration with an increased azotemia.
- Patients can be severely hyperkalemic.
- Urine specific gravity is high initially because the kidneys have lost their ability to concentrate urine. If obstruction continues long enough, permanent damage can occur and USG can lower (poor prognosis).
- If caught in the early phase, azotemia can revert to normal levels after urinary obstruction is removed and hydration is restored.

Secondary Concerns of Renal Disease

There are a number of secondary concerns that can occur when glomerular filtration is affected. Most concerns occur with chronic disease (i.e., chronic renal disease), as glomerular filtration and the ability to concentrate decrease over time. All secondary disease concerns should be evaluated when monitoring and treating a renal patient. Many secondary problems can make the patient worse if the medical team does not evaluate each component and treat accordingly. The following sections discuss these concerns.

Chronic Nonregenerative Anemia

Normal renal tissue produces a hormone called erythropoietin, which stimulates red blood cell formation from the bone marrow. With chronic kidney disease, erythropoietin levels decrease. This decreases red blood cell formation chronically and can produce moderate to severe anemia (Figure 5.9).

When treating the chronic kidney failure patient, the animal may present both anemic and dehydrated. As discussed in Chapter 2, this can produce a packed cell volume that may appear within low normal limits. As the medical team treats the renal patient with large amounts of intravenous fluids, blood fluid levels can return to normal or even produce a dilution effect on the red blood cell. This can produce patients with a life-threatening anemia within a few hours after the beginning of intravenous fluids (Figure 5.10).

Electrolyte Abnormalities

Sodium and potassium levels are responsible for producing electrical activity in the body. Sodium is a charged particle that is largely extracellular in the body. Potassium is a charged particle that is largely intracellular in the body. Sodium and potassium change places in order to create electrical

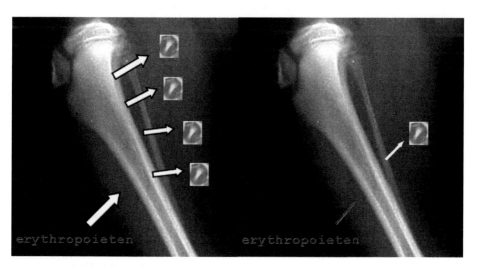

Figure 5.9. Illustration of how erthypoiten stimulates red blood cell production from the bone marrow (left). With chronic kidney disease, decreasing erythropoietin levels can produce a moderate to profound anemia (right).

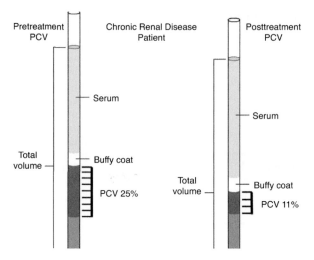

Figure 5.10. Illustration of how packed cell volume is affected by renal patients that are both dehydrated and anemic. The PCV on the left represents a cat with chronic renal failure prior to treatment. The PCV on the right represents the same patient after 6 hours of heavy fluid therapy.

current to produce muscular contractions, heartbeats, firing of neurons, and other body functions (Figure 5.11).

As discussed previously, chronic renal failure can produce chronic hypokalemia. Mild changes in hypokalemia can produce weakness, anorexia, and lethargy. In severe cases, a patient can become so weak that it cannot lift its head (ventroflexion of the neck; Figure 5.12).

Hypertension

The kidneys must preserve normal blood pressure to ensure that 20% of the blood is filtered by the kidney. As blood pressure decreases glomerular filtration also decreases, and over time the kidneys can deteriorate. To help prevent a decrease in blood volume, the kidneys use the renin-angiotensin system to increases blood

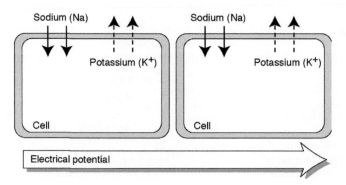

Figure 5.11. Illustration of how the exchange of sodium and potassium into and out of the cell body produces electrical energy for the body.

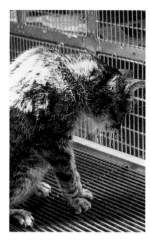

Figure 5.12. Ventroflexion of the neck: The body's potassium is so low that the patient cannot lift its neck.

pressure (Figure 5.13). There are specialized cells present within the arterioles of the glomeruli called juxtaglomerular cells, which stretch depending on blood pressure. As blood pressure decreases, the juxtaglomerular cells shrink, which stimulates the release of a chemical called renin. Renin activates another hormone called angiotensin → angiotensin I, which is produced by the liver. Then angiotensin I is changed into angiotensin II within the lungs. Angiotensin II is a potent constrictor of blood vessels, producing a whole body arteriole constriction. With increased constriction of the blood vessels, blood pressure rises, increasing blood through the kidneys and increasing glomerular filtration.

With patients suffering from chronic renal disease, the diseased tissue can still secrete renin even though 66–75% of both kidney tissues have been damaged or destroyed. As glomeruli begin to fail and their ability to filter blood is compromised, renin secretion increases. This continued process over time can produce constant hypertension.

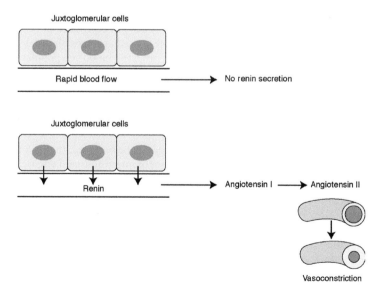

Figure 5.13. Illustration of the juxtaglomerular cells releasing renin in response to decreasing blood pressure. Renin activates angiotensin, a potent vasoconstrictor, increasing blood pressure.

Protein-Losing Nephropathy

As discussed previously, some forms of glomerular disease can produce damage to the glomerular filters, allowing larger molecules such as albumin to pass into the urinary space (see Figure 5.5). Over time, chronic blood protein levels decrease, producing **hypoalbuminemia**. Without normal blood albumin levels the body cannot heal properly and the patient can become weakened and anorexic. Further, albumin exerts a pressure on the fluid component of the blood (**oncotic pressure**) pulling fluid from the tissue into the blood so that the large protein molecule can be moved through the vascular supply. The hypoalbuminemic patient loses oncotic pressure and begins to push fluid from the blood supply back to the tissue, increasing the chances of fluid buildup in the tissues and lungs. Chronic renal patients that are hypoalbuminemic have an increased chance of fluid overload because fluid is more likely to move from the blood supply into the lungs.

Metabolic Acidosis

There are millions of chemical reactions that the body uses every day to produce energy, manufacture proteins, maintain normal homeostasis, and meet other daily needs (see Chapter 7). **All these reactions require a specific blood pH between 7.35–7.45. If the blood pH alters from this range, these reactions are slowed or do not occur.** With patients suffering from renal disease, loss of glomerular filtration, buildup of body toxins, and vomiting and diarrhea can occur. These factors can produce a blood pH <7.35, causing a metabolic acidosis; this can further produce weakness, anorexia, vomiting, and diarrhea, and the patient can develop shock.

Urogenital Diagnostic Tests

Because renal disease can develop as a subtle process and because kidney enzyme elevation can be seen with other disease conditions (e.g., dehydration, urinary obstruction), a full diagnostic workup can be indicated. The following sections present an overview of suggested clinical diagnostics.

Complete Blood Count

The complete blood count allows the veterinarian to determine changes in the red and white blood cell populations that can be affected by renal disease. Some changes that can be noted are reviewed in the following sections.

Changes in the Red Blood Cell Count

Chronic dehydration can cause an increased packed cell volume secondary to an acute or chronic disease. Pets that cannot concentrate their urine produce large amounts of dilute urine that can result in dehydration. A decreased red blood cell population/anemia also can occur secondarily to chronic decrease in erythropoietin levels.

Changes in the White Blood Cell Count

There can be bacterial, fungal, or protozoal causes of infectious renal disease, which can produce significant elevations of the white blood cell populations.

Blood Chemistry

As described previously, elevations in creatinine, BUN, and phosphorus and changes in electrolytes can all support the diagnosis of potential azotemia.

Urinalysis

Urinalysis is one of the most important clinical tests in defining renal disease and identifying early changes in kidney function. Evaluation of urine specific gravity in the azotemic patient confirms renal azotemia in most cases (see Chapter 9). The presence of protein in the urine may be an early indication of glomerular disease before the patient develops significant azotemia. Evaluating the **urinary sediment** for abnormality in cellular cytology can suggest the evidence of renal casts, white blood cells, urinary crystals, or abnormal cells, indicating disease of the bladder, kidneys, or reproductive organs (e.g., prostate).

Urine Culture and Sensitivity

If a heavy bacterial presence is noted in the urine in conjunction with increased urinary white blood cell count and renal casts (especially white blood cell casts), a urine culture and sensitivity should be considered (see chapter 9).

Urine Protein/Creatinine Ratio

If true renal proteinuria is detected (see Chapter 9) in a patient without obvious azotemia, an evaluation of urine protein/creatinine should be made. In most healthy patients, there should be a very small amount of protein in the urine compared to a large level or renal excreted creatinine; therefore, this ratio should be <1. As glomerular disease progresses, larger amounts of blood albumin will seep into the urine, increasing this ratio close to and beyond 1. Increasing ratio levels suggest more severe glomerular disease and help the medical team recognize affected kidneys and begin treatment before azotemia and severe weight loss occur.

Blood Pressure Monitoring

Because high blood pressure (hypertension) is a common secondary sequelae to renal disease, monitoring blood pressure with Doppler or oscillation equipment is strongly recommended. Screening ill patients before beginning large amounts of fluid therapy will decrease the risk of a worsening hypertension and development of retinal hemorrhage, cardiac enlargement, fluid overload, and death.

Blood Gas

Because loss of renal function can decrease renal perfusion, increase blood toxin, and produce diarrhea and vomiting, which can cause the loss of bicarbonate rich fluids, metabolic acidosis is a common secondary concern to renal patients. In evaluating blood gas (see chapter 12), the veterinarian can get a prognostic indicator of how severely affected the patient is and, with successive evaluation, monitor response to treatment.

Ethylene Glycol Test

If within the previous 8 hours antifreeze intoxication is suspected, an ethylene glycol test can help confirm whether ethylene glycol is evident in the body.

Abdominal Radiography

Radiographs of the abdomen can help the medical team evaluate kidney size and shape, determine whether there is evidence of renal or bladder stones, or note other abdominal organ changes that may suggest disease.

Abdominal Ultrasound

Abdominal ultrasound can help the medical team image the internal architecture of the abdominal organs to see changes in soft tissue suggestive of glomerular or medullary disease and determine the presence of stones or soft tissue calcification or the evidence of masses or tumors.

Through proper monitoring and evaluation of middle age to senior patients, renal disease can be detected early, its disease progression slowed, and secondary disease concerns can be monitored for and controlled. All members of the medical team must be able to understand the clinical diagnostics of renal disease, how to monitor for secondary concerns, and how to explain the disease and its concerns to the client.

Liver Physiology and Anatomy, Clinical Diagnostics, and Disease

As opposed to clinical diagnostic evaluation of renal disease and kidney function, the ability to evaluate liver damage vs. hepatic function is much more complex. This chapter reviews the changes in liver enzymes that are present in patients with liver trauma. However, note that changes in enzymes do not always mean that the liver is nonfunctional. **The other concern is that a patient can have severe debilitating liver disease with poor function and can still have blood work parameters within normal limits.** Team members must be able to understand the importance and the limitation of hepatic clinical diagnostics when approaching a patient with potential liver disease.

The liver sits in the cranial section of the abdomen on the right side of the body behind the diaphragm and caudal to the stomach and spleen (Figure 6.1).

The liver is divided into multiple lobes separated by fissures within the organ. In the canine and feline liver, the lobes are divided into the following:

- Left lateral lobe
- Left medial lobe
- Right lateral lobe
- Right medial lobe
- Quadrate lobe
- Caudate lobes

The liver also contains the **gallbladder,** which is the collecting site for deactivated toxins. The gallbladder is stimulated to contract, emptying its content through the common bile where it also shares ducts from the pancreas (see Chapter 7) before it empties into **the duodenum.** The ingestion of food and water stimulate the release of the pancreatic enzymes and constriction of the gallbladder through the common bile duct. Many of the toxins deactivated by the liver are color pigments (see the section "Bilirubin" below), which give the feces most of its color. Loss of liver function or obstruction of the gallbladder can produce retrograde flow of these bile pigments into the serum and tissue producing a yellow coloration (**icterus or jaundice**). Because bilirubin is a toxin, increased levels can make the patient weak, lethargic, and anorexic and produce vomiting and diarrhea.

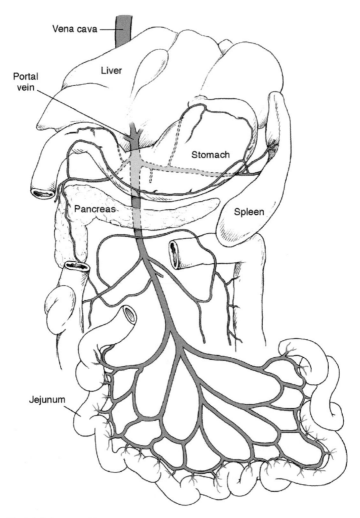

Figure 6.1.   Cranial abdomen architecture.

The liver has many functions in the body; the most important is detoxification of toxins. The small intestine absorbs all food stuff, microbes, and toxins into a large venous system called the **portal venous system.** The large portal vein carries all of these substances into the liver where intracellular chemicals (enzymes) detoxify toxins into inert waste products.

For the liver to be able to detoxify blood, the internal architecture of the liver must be adapted to filter blood, harvesting necessary nutrients and removing toxins. To do this, the liver architecture is divided into sinusoids where layers one cell thick of hepatocytes filter blood flowing from the portal vein to the hepatic central vein (Figure 6.2).

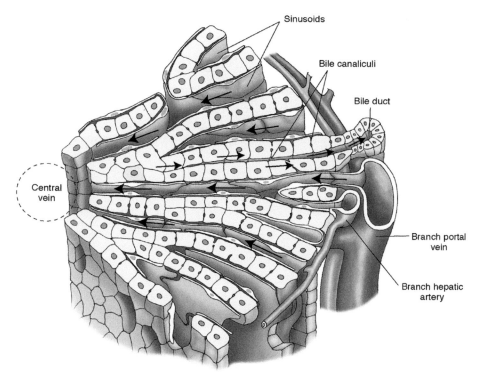

Sinusoids

Bile canaliculi

Bile duct

Central vein

Branch portal vein

Branch hepatic artery

Figure 6.2. A cross section of the hepatic sinusoid. A small branch of the portal vein passes through the tissue pushing blood into the central vein. Blood toxins, nutrients, and microbes are absorbed by the liver cells lining this sinus (**hepatocytes**). The toxins and microbes are deactivated and then pushed into a duct system called **bile canaliculi**, which then move the toxins into the gallbladder.

The function of these cells is to absorb all toxins, bacteria, and nutrients that are in the portal blood supply. The nutrients are absorbed, altered into other proteins, energy, and fats needed by the body and then released back into the blood venous flow for general circulation. The toxins and bacteria are deactivated and then released into channels, called **canaliculi**, running between layers of hepatocytes. These canaliculi lead to the bile ductules, which then move all deactivated sludge and debris into the gallbladder.

If the body is unable to detoxify these compounds, the active toxins can build up into the bloodstream and tissues. This can produce anorexia, weakness, weight loss, vomiting, and diarrhea. Further specific toxins can penetrate the central nervous system producing neurologic symptoms such as seizures, acute blindness, circling, head pressing, and abnormal behavior. Neurologic symptoms produced secondary to decreased hepatic function are called **hepatic encephalopathy.** Because this process is stimulated by the absorption of nutrients and improper detoxification of toxins, neurologic signs can be closely associated with feeding.

The liver also stores a small amount of a carbohydrate molecule called **glycogen.** Glycogen is broken down into sugar when the blood sugar stores rapidly decrease and fat has not yet been mobilized.

Table 6.1.   Risks of patients with reduced hepatic function.

Liver Function	Concern of Dysfunction
Detoxification	*Hepatic encephalopathy*: Neurologic symptoms develop secondary to improper detoxification of microbes and toxins, which remain in the body affecting the central nervous system.
	Physical symptoms due to build of toxins and bilirubin: Increased toxins can produce nausea, anorexia, depression, vomiting, diarrhea, weakness, and weight loss
Formation of building blocks	*Anemia*: Lack of red blood cell precursors
	Increased clotting time: The liver produces clotting factors that finalize clot formation.
	Hypoalbuminemia: Due to lack of blood albumin, the body can shift fluid from the vascular supply to the tissue, increasing fluid accumulation in the body, producing ascites, edema, and pulmonary edema (with patients on IV fluids).
Glucose storage	*Hypoglycemia* (rare)

Finally, the liver produces many of the body's building blocks necessary for normal maintenance, growth, and production. It is important to note that the liver produces many of the necessary components needed for red blood cell production and clotting factors (see Chapter 13). Therefore, animals with chronic hepatic disease may develop chronic anemia and may have decreased ability to clot blood. **With this concern, no jugular blood collection should ever be attempted with patients suffering from potential hepatic disease or dysfunction.**

The liver also produces a protein molecule called **albumin.** Albumin's function is to carry other molecules and hormones around the bloodstream in a deactivated form until the body requires the chemical. In order to move albumin through the bloodstream, large amounts of fluid must be pulled from the tissue. This physiological draw of fluid that albumin exerts on the tissue is called **oncotic pressure.** Loss of albumin production secondary to liver dysfunction can decrease oncotic pressure, increasing the amount of fluid returning to the tissue. If severe, large amounts of fluid accumulation can occur within the abdomen (**ascites**). Medical team members must be extremely cautious with hospitalized patients with low albumin levels on intravenous fluids because these patients have increased risk of pushing larger amounts of fluids into the tissue. This increases risks of moving fluid into lung tissue producing pulmonary edema and developing fluid overload (Table 6.1).

Diseases of the Liver

Liver disease can take many forms, and unlike renal disease, where general treatment options include fluid therapy, medications, and hospitalization, medical and surgical therapy can be extremely variable dependent on the type of liver disease present. In many cases, final diagnosis of liver disease must be based on liver biopsy.

Infectious Liver Disease

Viral, bacterial, fungal, and parasitic pathogens can infect and invade normal liver tissue, producing acute or chronic disease and debilitation.

Inflammatory Disease

Hepatitis is the activation of the immune system by some foreign antigen within the liver. This antigenic stimulation produces an influx of white blood cells through a healthy liver, causing damage and irritation. Inflammatory disease can be acute, chronic, or end-stage (**cirrhosis**).

Cancer (Neoplasia)

The liver is both the site of primary cancer and a common site of secondary metastatic disease (Figure 6.3). Some common cancers that primarily affect the liver are hepatic adenocarcinoma, hepatic cholangioadenocarcinoma, lymphoma, and mast cell tumor.

Metabolic Disease

This form of liver disease occurs as inert compounds buildup within the liver, destroying the normal architecture and liver function. Common metabolic diseases of the liver include hepatic lipidosis and amyloidosis (protein).

Hepatic Lipidosis

This disease syndrome occurs commonly in the cat and horse (pony) when these ani-

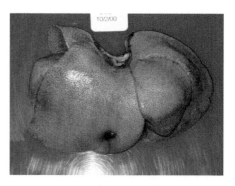

Figure 6.4. Image of a liver) infiltrated by large amounts of fat (hepatic lipidosis).

mals have a disease entity that produces a profound anorexia. The animals shunt large amounts of fat into the liver to transform it into sugar. The movement of fat into the liver is so severe that normal liver architecture and liver function can be affected (Figure 6.4).

Amyloidosis (Protein)

Amyloidosis is an accumulation of an inert protein in the liver, which can chronically destroy normal liver tissue. The buildup of this abnormal protein is most commonly seen in the shar-pei breed, in which amyloidosis can be associated with kidney and liver disease and inflammatory changes in the joint capsule.

Toxin Disease

Because the liver is the major detoxifying organ in the body, toxins can damage normal liver tissue, which affects function.

Portacaval Shunts

In some patients, a small blood vessel, called a shunt, can occur from the portal vein to the caudal vena cava, producing a bypass of blood flow around the liver.

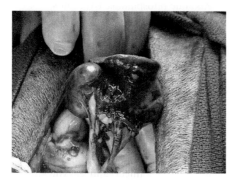

Figure 6.3. Image of a liver with primary cancer or metastasis.

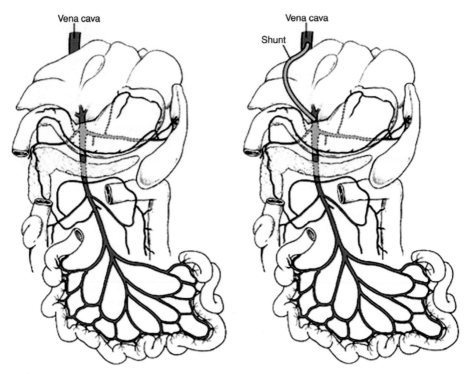

Figure 6.5. Illustration of an extrahepatic shunt. In the figure on the left, the portal vein courses normally into the liver. In the illustration on the right, there is a small vessel that bypasses the liver (shunt) allowing the movement of toxins into normal circulation prior to liver metabolism.

In these patients, blood toxins bypass the liver and enter the general bloodstream and produce severe neurological and systemic signs. Shunts can occur as a congenital defect or as an acquired disease and can occur within the liver (intrahepatic) or outside of the liver (extrahepatic) (Figure 6.5).

Identifying Liver Damage vs. Hepatic Dysfunction

Within the liver cells are enzymes that function to change or produce specific body-building blocks or detoxify toxic chemicals in the body. Clinically, we evaluate the following intracellular enzymes:

- Alanine aminotransferase (ALT)
- Aspartate aminotransferase (AST)
- Gamma-glutamyltransferase (GGT)
- Alkaline phosphatase (Alk Phos)

Unlike evaluating kidney disease by monitoring azotemia (see Chapter 5), these clinical diagnostics do not represent a buildup of toxin but rather normal enzymes produced within the hepatocytes. Normally, a specific level of each enzyme leaks from the hepatocyte into the bloodstream. Acute trauma to hepatocytes can produce sharp elevations of liver enzymes by leakage of enzymes out of the damaged hepatocyte into the blood or by increased production of enzymes from chronic stimulation or irritation. **Increases in these liver enzymes support liver trauma,** but they do not always suggest liver dysfunction. However, with chronic to end-stage disease, there may enough hepatic enzymes within the bloodstream to produce normal blood levels in clinical testing, but the liver may not be functional.

Hepatocytes also produce chemicals called **bile acids** that help to emulsify fat within the small intestine. Bile acids are stimulated when the patient eats. Bile acids then empty through the gallbladder and into the common bile duct. After fat is emulsified, bile acids are then rapidly reabsorbed by the small intestine.

Clinical Diagnostics That Identify Acute Liver Damage

Alanine Aminotransferase (ALT)

Alanine aminotransferase (ALT) is responsible for the conversion of 2-oxoglutarate to pyruvate and glutamate in the liver cells (hepatocytes). Although blood levels of alanine aminotransferase can vary from lab to lab, normal ALT levels are generally as shown in Chart 6.1.

Chart 6.1

Canine	50–60 IU/L
Feline	28–76 IU/L

The following sections review patterns in the ALT level.

Low ALT Activity

Low ALT activity is not generally associated with disease conditions.

Increased Activity of the Enzyme

Increased activity of the enzyme in the blood occurs when there are alterations in the lipid membrane of the hepatocytes,

secondary to injury, inflammations, or infection within the liver. The increased blood levels do not indicate the severity of the damage to the hepatocytes or degree of reversibility of the disease process. Further ALT activity can also be increased secondary to the following:

- Chronic use of anticonvulsants, steroids, and other drugs
- Physical trauma
- Cardiac disease

Aspartate Aminotransferase (AST or SGOT)

Aspartate aminotransferase (AST) is an intracellular enzyme in all cells, but it has higher levels of activity in muscle and liver cell damage. Although blood levels of aspartate aminotransferase can vary from lab to lab, normal AST levels generally are as shown in Chart 6.2.

Chart 6.2

Canine	5–55 IU/L
Feline	5–55 IU/L

The following sections review patterns in the AST level.

Decreased AST Activity

Low ALT activity is not generally associated with disease conditions.

Increased AST Activity

As with ALT, AST blood levels in the blood occur when there are alterations in the lipid membrane of the hepatocytes, secondary to injury, inflammations, or infection within the liver. The increased blood levels do not indicate the severity of the damage to the hepatocytes or degree of reversibility of the disease process. Further AST activity can also be increased secondary to the following:

- Disease that affects the muscular skeletal system (e.g., trauma or seizure)
- Disease that produces red blood cell destruction (e.g., immune-mediated hemolytic anemia) because there are significant levels of AST in red blood cells.

Gamma-glutamyltransferase (GGT)

Gamma-glutamyltransferase is more an indicator of gallbladder obstruction or lack of bile flow. GGT is an intracellular enzyme responsible for cleaving C-terminal glutamyl groups from one substrate or molecule to another, and it is thought to be involved in pathways used to protect cells from oxidative injury. GGT is present in all cells except that it has higher concentration in renal epithelial, bile duct, and hepatic cells. Although blood levels of gamma-glutamyltransferase can vary from lab to lab, normal GGT levels are generally as shown in Chart 6.3:

Chart 6.3

Canine	0–10 IU/L
Feline	1–7 IU/L

The following sections review patterns of GGT levels.

Decreased GGT Activity

Low GGT activity is not generally associated with disease conditions.

Elevations in GGT

Increased GGT activity can be associated with decreased bile flow (**cholestasis**). Further, GGT can increase with liver damage that produces cholestasis. Unlike AST and ALT, GGT does not "leak" from hepato-

cytes; its activity is increased due to increased production (**induction**) of the enzyme in response to disease.

Alkaline Phosphatase (SALP or ALP)

Alkaline phosphatase is present within the liver, intestine, bone, kidneys, and placenta. On most chemistry panels, alkaline phosphatase activity represents the combined activity of all combined tissue alkaline phosphatase levels. Although blood levels of alkaline phosphatase can vary from lab to lab, normal ALP levels are generally as shown in Chart 6.4.

Chart 6.4

Canine	10–150 IU/L
Feline	0–62 IU/L

The following sections review patterns of ALP.

Decreased ALP Activity

Low ALP activity is not generally associated with disease conditions.

Increased ALP Activity

High ALP can originate from diseases and nondiseased conditions. Similar to GGT, ALP's activity increases because of increased production of the enzyme (induction) in response to disease. The following are some conditions that increase ALP activity:

Hyperadrenocorticism. Although not a specific test for hyperadrenocorticism (Cushing's disease, see Chapter 11), chronic production of adrenal cortisol (steroid) increases production of alkaline phosphatase. Further, the administration of oral corticosteroids can cause increased ALP activity.

Liver and Gallbladder Disease. With chronic hepatic or gallbladder disease, increases in ALP production can be observed.

Long-term medication. Patients on specific long-term medication (e.g., phenobarbital, prednisone) can increase production of ALP.

Bone growth. Rapid changes in bone (e.g., growth, bone cancer) can increase blood levels of alkaline phosphatase from production within the bone.

Clinical Diagnostics That Identify Liver Dysfunction

Liver dysfunction is due to acute or chronic damage to liver tissue affecting normal production of liver compounds and hepatic detoxification. **Determining whether the disease is acute or chronic is not as important as determining whether there is hepatic trauma or, more importantly, hepatic dysfunction.** The following sections identify chemistry parameters that suggest liver dysfunction.

Bilirubin

Bilirubin is a toxic metabolite produced from the red blood cell destruction in the spleen and the breakdown of hemoglobin. As red blood cells age, they are removed from circulation in the spleen, lysed, and the iron molecule removed from the hemoglobin molecule to be used again. The remaining chemical is bilirubin, which is moved to the liver to be detoxified and excreted through the gallbladder. Although blood levels of bilirubin can vary from lab to lab, normal levels are generally as shown in Chart 6.5.

Chart 6.5

Canine	0.0–0.6 mg/dL
Feline	0.0–0.4 mg/dL

The buildup of bilirubin in the serum and body in association with liver disease indicates liver dysfunction. **However, it should be noted that although patients that are icteric secondary to liver disease have liver dysfunction, not all patients with liver dysfunction are icteric.** Furthermore, increased levels of bilirubin also can be associated with increased intravascular red blood cell destruction (e.g., immune-mediated hemolytic anemias) or gallbladder obstruction.

Blood Urea Nitrogen (BUN)

A low BUN level can be associated with the liver's inability to take ammonia molecules and produce BUN. When observed on clinical diagnostics, it may suggest a liver dysfunction. *A low BUN by itself does not always indicate liver dysfunction.* Low-protein diets can also result in a low BUN. Although blood levels of BUN can vary from lab to lab, normal BUN levels are generally as shown in Chart 6.6.

Chart 6.6

Canine	10–26 mg/dL
Feline	15–34 mg/dL

Albumin

As discussed previously, albumin is a small carrier protein that binds to hormones and other components in the bloodstream to maintain and move necessary elements throughout the body. Decreases in blood albumin concentration can occur generally with a number of disease syndromes that affect production or loss of the protein molecule. A decrease in functioning hepatocytes will compromise the liver's ability to produce albumin. As a general rule, at least 75% of normal liver function must be lost before albumin concentration is decreased.

When attributable to liver disease, hypoalbuminemia can be an indicator of altered liver function. However, low body albumin can also be associated with kidney disease (see Chapter 5), bleeding (see Chapter 14), and intestinal disease (see Chapter 7). Although blood levels of albumin can vary from lab to lab, normal albumin levels are generally as shown in Chart 6.7.

Chart 6.7

Canine	3.1–4.5 g/dL
Feline	2.4–4.1 g/dL

Bile Acids

As discussed previously, bile acids are excreted in response to eating to help emulsify fat. In liver disease, bile acids are not properly reabsorbed and represent a true liver dysfunction. To evaluate bile acids, the patient is fasted for 12 hours and a baseline level of bile acids are drawn. Then the animal is fed a high-energy food, and 2 hours later another bile acid level is collected. In an animal with liver dysfunction, prefeeding (preprandial) bile acids are high and postfeeding (postprandial) bile acids are even higher. Although bile acid levels can vary from lab to lab, normal levels are as shown in Chart 6.8.

Chart 6.8

Canine	Preprandial: 0–5 μmol/L Postprandial: <25 μmol/L
Feline	Preprandial: 0–5 μmol/L Postprandial: <15 μmol/L

Hepatic Clinical Diagnostics

Because liver disease, trauma, and dysfunction can be difficult to evaluate based on blood work alone, the medical team must also evaluate the history, physical examination, and other diagnostic aids. There are many potential forms of liver disease; blood work can appear normal and there can still be significant liver dysfunction. Further, clinical diagnostics and imaging alone are often not sufficient to diagnose the cause of the liver disease present. If the medical team determines that hepatic dysfunction is occurring, a liver biopsy (fine needle, tissue biopsy, or core biopsy) may be recommended to obtain a final diagnosis and help outline treatment protocols (Algorithm 6.1). Overall, a clinical diagnostic evaluation for a hepatic patient may include the tests described in the following sections.

Complete Blood Count

Components of the complete blood count can vary depending on the form of liver disease; however, general trends should be monitored for red blood cells, white blood cells, and platelets.

Red Blood Cells

With chronic waning disease, chronic anemia may be present secondary to the lack of precursors for cellular components. Chronic liver disease also can affect the patient's ability to clot blood. With significant anemia, platelet number, clotting times, and a blood film should be evaluated to determine whether the patient has a nonregenerative anemia vs. chronic bleeding concerns.

White Blood Cells

With concerns of infectious disease, changes in white blood cells should be evaluated. With certain forms of cancer (e.g., hepatic lymphoma), white blood cell elevations can be severe, with extremely abnormal cytology and high white blood cell. A blood smear is always suggested with sick animals to better assess cell morphology (red

Algorithm 6.1. Hepatic clinical diagnosis

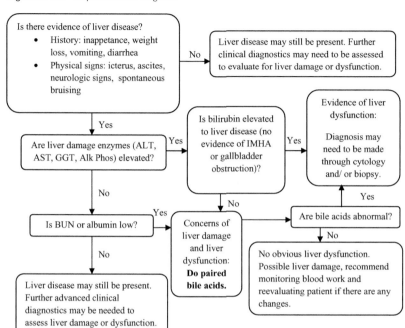

blood cells and white blood cells) as well as platelet numbers.

Platelets

With concerns of decreased clotting factors and an inability to finalize the clotting process (**coagulopathy**), platelets counts should also be closely monitored. **Animals should be carefully assessed for bruising, and jugular sticks should not be attempted if there is concern of a coagulopathy.**

Chemistry

As discussed previously, blood work on a routine chemistry can be extremely variable with acute or chronic liver disease, portacaval shunts, and neoplasia. The medical team's responsibility is to try to identify an-

imals with liver damage or chronic disease and try to assess hepatic function.

Coagulation Screen

Evaluating clotting times—**activated clotting time (ACT), partial thromboplastin time (PT), activated partial thromboplastin time (APTT)**—can help detect early trends of the patient's ability to clot blood (see Chapter 14).

Abdominal Radiography

Abdominal radiographs can help assess for changes in hepatic size and shape, evidence of gallbladder for stones (**cholelithe**), and any other changes in the abdomen that can suggest serious disease.

Abdominal Ultrasound

Abdominal ultrasound can assess the internal architecture of the abdominal organs for changes suggestive of focal or diffuse hepatic disease, changes in the gallbladder wall suggestive of infection or obstruction, and identification of abnormal blood vessels that could suggest a portacaval shunt. It is important to note that changes in hepatic architecture can only suggest focal or diffuse disease and rarely helps the medical team confirm diagnosis. Cellular or tissue biopsy is possible through ultrasound-guided biopsy techniques.

Exploratory Surgery

In some cases, when ultrasonic biopsy or fine needle aspirate is nondiagnostic, exploratory or laparoscopic surgery and wedge or core biopsy of the liver may be needed.

Pancreatic and Gastrointestinal Physiology and Anatomy, Clinical Diagnostics, and Disease

The gastrointestinal system is a tubular system running from the animal's mouth to its rectum (Figure 7.1). Several regions within this system have been specialized to help break down and absorb nutrients, reabsorb water, and excrete toxins produced by the kidneys and liver. The mouth, stomach, and early small intestine (e.g., duodenum and jejunum) function to break down the foodstuff and absorb nutrients. The lower intestine (ileum and large colon) is responsible for reabsorbing water, forming fecal material, and producing a source of water-soluble vitamins through fermentation in most domestic animals.

The clinical diagnostic testing of the gastrointestinal system is utilized when patients are having problems in digesting food (**maldigestion**) and absorbing nutrients (**malabsorption**) and with concerns of intestinal bleeding. As discussed previously, patients with concerns of chronic intestinal disease must be evaluated based on their history, physical exam, complete blood and urine diagnostics, fecal examinations, and advanced imaging (e.g., radiology or ultra-sonography). However, there are specific diagnostics indicated once intestinal disease has been identified.

Maldigestion/Malabsorption Syndrome

Patients that have decreased ability to digest and absorb nutrients often present with vomiting, weight loss, increased appetite, and soft cow-patty stools with or without the presence of thick, tarry, digested blood (**melena**). These patients can develop the following changes in their clinical diagnostics.

Albumin

As discussed previously, low body albumin (**hypoalbuminemia**) can occur secondary to bleeding, renal disease, and liver disease. Patients with malabsorption/maldigestion disease (e.g., inflammatory bowel disease, lymphangectasia, intestinal neoplasia) can have depletions in essential amino acids

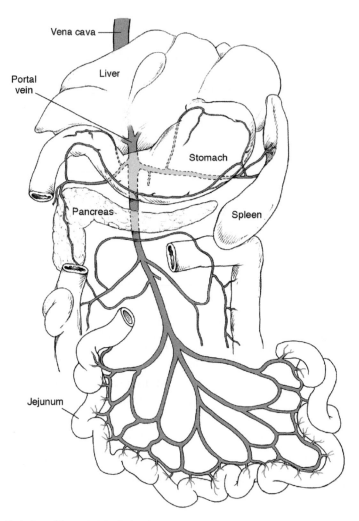

Figure 7.1. Illustration of the gastrointestinal system.

and proteins, producing hypoalbuminemia (**protein-losing enteropathy**). Patients with a persistently low albumin levels should be evaluated for chronic bleeding, renal loss, liver dysfunction, or chronic gastrointestinal disease. Although blood levels of albumin can vary from lab to lab, normal albumin levels are generally as shown in Chart 7.1.

Chart 7.1

Canine	3.1–4.5 g/dL
Feline	2.4–4.1 g/dL

Blood Folate Levels

Diseases that can affect chronic digestion can alter normal gastrointestinal bacterial populations and decrease normal bacterial fermentation. This change in bacterial populations can lead to overgrowth of other pathogenic bacteria, which can make gastrointestinal signs worse. Further, with chronic decreased bacterial fermentation and pathogenic bacteria overgrowth, the production of the B vitamin folate decreases. Low blood folate levels can help support the diagnosis of chronic intestinal disease. Although blood levels of folic acid can vary from lab to lab, normal levels are generally as shown in Chart 7.2.

Chart 7.2

Canine	6.5–11.5 ng/ml
Feline	9.7–21.6 ng/ml

Intestinal Bleeding

In patients that present with chronic tarry stool or blood vomiting (**hematemesis**), concerns of chronic intestinal ulceration and bleeding should be explored. Gastrointestinal ulceration can occur secondary to drug interactions (e.g., Nonsteroidal antiinflammatory drugs, steroids), ulcer formation, tumors, or diseases that produce chronic bleeding problems. To help determine whether the patient has chronic intestinal bleeding, the medical team should evaluate the diagnostics in the following sections.

Complete Blood Count and Blood Film

Patients with chronic intestinal bleeding present mildly anemic with evidence of regeneration in their blood film. Team members should evaluate blood films for nucleated red blood cells, reticulocytes, Howell-Jolly bodies, and polychromasia, which help to indicate that a regenerative anemia is occurring (Figure 7.2). It is important to note that the only true hallmark of regeneration is a reticulocyte count; the other changes noted above help to support evidence that a regenerative anemia is occurring. With chronic bleeding, a decreased platelet (**thrombocytopenia**) count may also be observed.

BUN and the BUN/Creatinine Ratio

Blood that accumulates in the intestine secondary to ulceration is digested and absorbed like any other nutrient. Digestion of red blood cells increases the amount of body ammonia, which then produces an increased BUN level (see Chapter 5). By comparing the amount of BUN to creatinine, this ratio can suggest an increased production of BUN that is not associated with glomerular filtration. An elevation in this ratio is not an absolute indication of intestinal bleeding because other factors may also increase BUN (e.g., high-protein meals) without affecting creatinine levels.

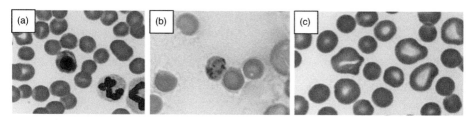

Figure 7.2.   Evidence of a regenerative anemia: (**a**) nucleated red blood cells, (**b**) reticulocytes, (**c**) polychromasia.

Albumin

As discussed previously, hypoalbuminemia can also be observed with chronic bleeding.

The pancreas sits in the cranial abdomen. The right lobe lays lateral to the duodenum extending from the middle part of the right kidney to the pyloric region of the stomach. The left lobe lays caudal to the stomach and perpendicular to the duodenum (see Figure 7.1). The pancreas functions both as an exocrine and endocrine organ. Exocrine glands, which play an important part in normal body functions (i.e., salivary gland, sweat gland, mammary gland), secrete chemicals through a duct network. The pancreas secretes two enzymes, **lipase** and **amylase**, that aid in the breakdown of foodstuff. Amylase cleaves large sugar molecules into smaller single sugars. Lipase breaks down fat into smaller molecules so that they can be absorbed by the intestine. Lipase and amylase are produced in response to ingestion of food and water and production of hydrochloric acid by the stomach. Both enzymes are critical to the digestive process.

Endocrine glands secrete hormones directly into the bloodstream that affect other organs in the body (i.e., pituitary, thyroid, sex organs). The endocrine pancreas produces **insulin** and **glucagon**, which help maintain normal blood sugar levels. Insulin is released in times of increasing blood sugar to stimulate the conversion of sugar into glycogen (liver) and fat. Glucagon is produced in response to lower blood sugar levels to stimulate the conversion of glycogen and fat back into glucose. Insulin and glucagon are produced by specialized regions of cells called the **islets of Langerhans** (Figure 7.3).

Pancreatic disease can affect both the exocrine or endocrine components of the pancreas. Common pancreatic exocrine diseases are reviewed in the following sections.

Pancreas

Pancreatitis

Pancreatitis is an inflammation or infection of the pancreas, producing a leakage of lipase and amylase onto the organ surface. The release of these enzymes begins an autodigestion of the pancreas resulting in worsening inflammation, severe whole body illness, and the potential for secondary organ disease (e.g., kidney and liver) and infection (sepsis). Classically, patients present with extremely painful abdomens, experiencing vomiting and diarrhea, and severely dehydrated. Further, if the swelling is severe, the gallbladder ducts that empty through the pancreas and into the small intestine can become obstructed, producing jaundice and secondary hepatic disease.

Pancreatic Exocrine Insufficiency (PEI)

PEI is a rare congenital or acquired disease of the acinar cells resulting in a lack of production of exocrine pancreatic enzymes. These animals suffer from a severe malabsorption/maldigestion syndrome because they are not able to digest normal nutrients. Patients usually appear very happy and energetic, but are very thin with decreased muscle mass, are always hungry, and have severe cow-patty diarrhea. The congenital disease is seen most commonly in the German shepherd breed. The acquired disease can often occur after severe chronic destructive pancreatitis.

Pancreatic Tumors

Pancreatic tumors are rarely seen in the feline and canine, closely mimicking pancreatitis. Patients present with chronic vomiting and diarrhea, abdominal tenderness, dehydration, and depression.

As with liver disease, clinical diagnostic blood work is a large part of the diagnostic protocol; however, in the case of

Algorithm 7.1. Clinical diagnostics of the gastrointestinal system.

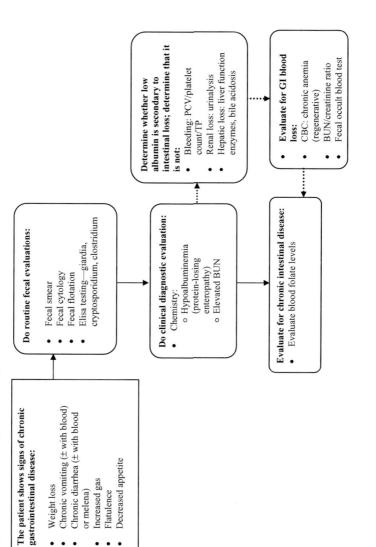

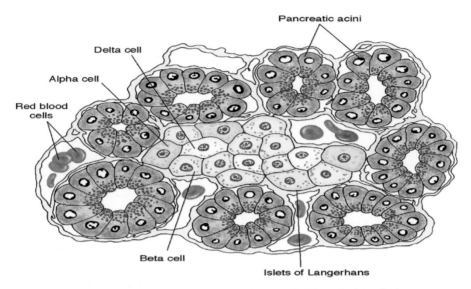

Figure 7.3. Small section of the pancreas showing the pancreatic acinar cells, which produce lipase and amylase (exocrine) and the islet of Langerhans (endocrine), which produces insulin and glucagon.

pancreatitis, baseline blood work may not indicate the severity of the syndrome and **often blood work is nonconclusive.** Clinical diagnostics for the exocrine pancreas can include those reviewed in the following sections.

Complete Blood Count

Dependent on the disease and its acuteness or chronicity, changes in the complete blood count can be variable. The following sections review changes that can be noticed.

Pancreatitis

With acute disease, dehydration can produce elevation in the red blood cell count. Further, secondary to inflammation or infection, elevations in the white blood cell count can be observed. As discussed previously, team members should evaluate blood smears for increased numbers of immature neutrophils (bands). These patients can have a normal white blood cell count initially, but the increase in bands can reflect acute inflammatory or infectious changes (Figure 7.4). With chronic exocrine pancreatic disease, the complete blood count can be normal.

Pancreatic Exocrine Insufficiency

Generally, the complete blood count can be normal with patients who have PEI.

Pancreatic Tumor

Animals with pancreatic tumors may produce chronic (nonregenerative) anemia due to the progressive disease consuming precursors necessary to produce normal red blood cells (**anemia of chronic disease**).

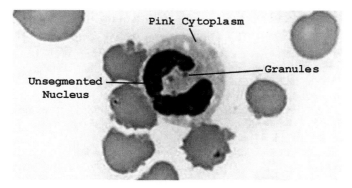

Figure 7.4. Image of an immature neutrophil (band). Band neutrophils can be identified by their unsegmented nucleus, pink cytoplasm, and evident vacuoles. Increasing levels of band neutrophils can suggest massive whole body infection even before increases in the total white blood cell count.

Clinical Chemistry

With pancreatic exocrine disease, patients may have severe disease evident, and changes in the blood chemistry can be normal.

Pancreatitis

Canine

Evaluate the serum. Team members should begin by evaluating for the presence of lipemia, which can suggest altered fat metabolism.

Amylase. Increased serum amylase can be a suggestive indicator of acute pancreatitis is the canine. **It is not helpful in evaluation of feline pancreatitis.** Although blood levels of amylase can vary from lab to lab, normal levels are generally as shown in Chart 7.3.

Chart 7.3

Canine	500–1500 IU/L
Feline	500–1500 IU/L

Lipase. Increased serum lipase can be a suggestive indicator of acute pancreatitis is the canine. **It is not helpful in evaluation** of feline pancreatitis. Although blood levels of Lipase can vary from lab to lab, normal levels are generally as shown in Chart 7.4.

Chart 7.4

Canine	10–500 IU/L
Feline	10–195 IU/L

Feline

Blood chemistry and serum can be completely normal even with severe disease.

Pancreatic Insufficiency

Chemistry results are generally within normal listed parameters.

Pancreatic Tumor

With the concern of pancreatic cancer, lipase and amylase may show significant elevations in the routine chemistry. **It is important to note that a normal lipase and amylase level do not rule out the possibility of pancreatic cancer.**

Trypsinlike Immunoassay (TLI)

TLI is a blood test that allows the medical team to assess the levels of trypsin, a proteolytic enzyme in the body that is activated by normal pancreatic activity. In the canine, increased TLI levels can be suggestive of chronic pancreatitis or pancreatic cancer. In the canine, decreased TLI levels suggest lack of lipase and amylase production strongly indicating PEI.

Canine Pancreatic Lipase Inhibition Test (cPLI)

The cPLI is used as a screening test for pancreatitis. Pancreatic lipase inhibitor levels increase dramatically, suggesting that pancreatic inflammation and irritation are occurring. There are no noted changes in cPLI levels with PEI or pancreatic tumor.

Blood Folate Levels

As discussed previously, decreasing levels of folate can suggest alteration in normal bacterial synthesis in the gastrointestinal system, which can support a chronic inflammation of the pancreas and gastrointestinal system. This test is often used with other clinical diagnostic test to help confirm chronic pancreatitis.

Radiology

Although difficult to interpret with abdominal radiographs, appearance of the pancreatic region and position of the duodenum may suggest enlargement of the pancreas due to inflammation or secondary infections.

Ultrasound

Ultrasound studies of the pancreatic region are an important diagnostic indicated in evaluating changes in the pancreas that suggest disease, abscess, or cancer. Further, ultrasound-guided fine needle aspirates can be helpful in identifying pancreatic disease.

Secondary disease concerns due to diseases of the exocrine pancreas occur largely as a result of severe chronic or acute pancreatitis. With pancreatitis, the severe whole body inflammation and possible secondary infection can produce conditions reviewed in the following sections (see Algorithm 7.2).

Renal Failure

Renal damage occurs as dehydration from pancreatitis produces decreased blood flow through the kidneys, producing hypotension and decreased glomerular filtration. Decreased glomerular filtration (see Chapter 5) causes a worsening azotemia and worsens dehydration, which can develop into an acute renal failure.

Gallbladder Obstruction

With severe swelling or infection of the pancreas, the bile ducts, which empty into the intestine through the pancreas, can be occluded. The patient will start to become icteric and weak as toxins from the gallbladder cannot empty into the small intestine. This change signifies a worsening in the condition and prognosis.

Hepatic Failure

Continued dehydration, decreased blood flow, and potential secondary ascending

Algorithm 7.2. Acute exocrine pancreatic patient (pancreatitis)—canine.

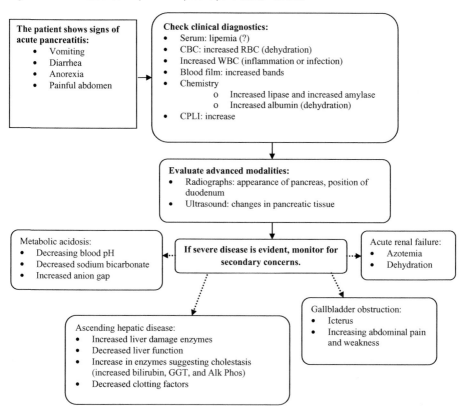

infection from the pancreas can produce a secondary hepatitis. Acute hepatic dysfunction can lead to decreased clotting factors, an inability to detoxify toxins, and decreased bacterial clearance.

Metabolic Acidosis

The loss of normal glomerular filtration, increased body toxins, and vomiting and diarrhea that can occur with pancreatitis can develop a serious metabolic acidosis (see

Chapter 12). Clinically, team members will identify metabolic acidosis by observing a change in blood pH (pH < 7.25), a normal or decreased partial pressure of carbon dioxide (pCO_2), decreasing levels of blood bicarbonate levels, and a decreasing base excess.

With chronic pancreatic disease, chronic destruction of the pancreas can produce destruction of either exocrine or endocrine tissue. The following sections review diseases that can occur secondary to chronic pancreatic disease (see Algorithms 7.3 & 7.4).

Algorithm 7.3. Chronic exocrine pancreatic patient (pancreatitis)—canine.

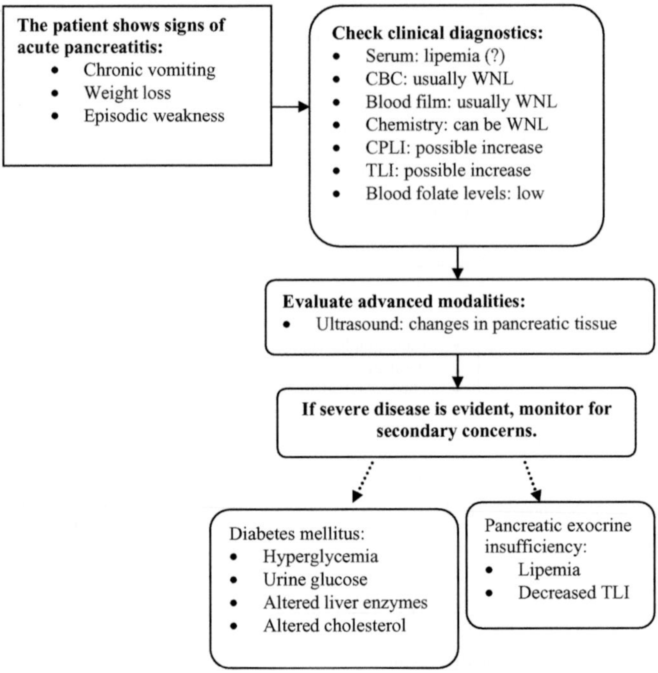

The patient shows signs of acute pancreatitis:
- Chronic vomiting
- Weight loss
- Episodic weakness

Check clinical diagnostics:
- Serum: lipemia (?)
- CBC: usually WNL
- Blood film: usually WNL
- Chemistry: can be WNL
- CPLI: possible increase
- TLI: possible increase
- Blood folate levels: low

Evaluate advanced modalities:
- Ultrasound: changes in pancreatic tissue

If severe disease is evident, monitor for secondary concerns.

Diabetes mellitus:
- Hyperglycemia
- Urine glucose
- Altered liver enzymes
- Altered cholesterol

Pancreatic exocrine insufficiency:
- Lipemia
- Decreased TLI

Diabetes Mellitus—Endocrine Disease of the Pancreas

Disease of the endocrine pancreas results from loss of production of or lack of tissue response to insulin-producing diabetes mellitus. There are three potential causes of diabetes mellitus in the canine and feline.

Type I Diabetes

Type I diabetes results from a lack of insulin production causing increased glucose levels and, in some cases, ketone production. As insulin levels decrease, the patient tries to remove the excess sugar by excreting it in the urine and transforming it into fat metabolically. The increased demand for fat production overwhelms the chemical intermediaries necessary, and the body can produce only a chemical toxin called **acetone,** which is a ketone. Type I Diabetes is due to exhaustion of the islet cells and is seen more commonly in canines and obese animals.

Type II Diabetes

Type II Diabetes is produced by an insulin resistance by peripheral tissue, slowed production of insulin, or decreased production of insulin. Insulin has decreased

Algorithm 7.4. Acute/chronic exocrine pancreatic patient (pancreatitis)—feline.

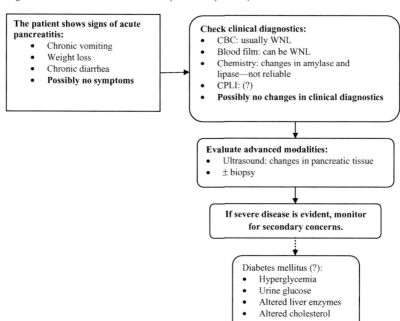

The patient shows signs of acute pancreatitis:
- Chronic vomiting
- Weight loss
- Chronic diarrhea
- **Possibly no symptoms**

Check clinical diagnostics:
- CBC: usually WNL
- Blood film: can be WNL
- Chemistry: changes in amylase and lipase—not reliable
- CPLI: (?)
- **Possibly no changes in clinical diagnostics**

Evaluate advanced modalities:
- Ultrasound: changes in pancreatic tissue
- ± biopsy

If severe disease is evident, monitor for secondary concerns.

Diabetes mellitus (?):
- Hyperglycemia
- Urine glucose
- Altered liver enzymes
- Altered cholesterol

effect on peripheral tissue producing hyperglycemia, but typically this form is not severe enough to produce ketones. This syndrome is much more common in felines and if continued chronically enough, these patients can become Type I diabetics.

Type III Diabetes

This type of diabetes is secondary to a primary underlying disease. Common diseases that can produce diabetes mellitus are chronic pancreatitis, hyperadrenocorticism (Cushing's disease), hyperthyroidism, and animals on specific prolonged drug therapy (e.g., estrogens, steroids).

Clinical diagnostics to determine whether diabetes is evident in the patient are largely focused on blood and urine samples. Clinical diagnostic changes in the diabetic patient are reviewed in the following sections (see Algorithm 7.5).

Complete Blood Count

Typically in diabetic animals, there are no overall changes in complete blood count.

Chemistry

Serum

Due to decreased ability to move sugar into fat, many patients will have chronic lipemic serum.

Algorithm 7.5. Endocrine pancreatic patient (Diabetes mellitus).

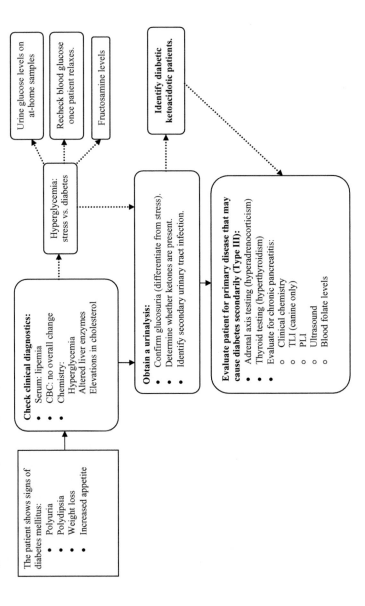

The patient shows signs of diabetes mellitus:
- Polyuria
- Polydipsia
- Weight loss
- Increased appetite

Check clinical diagnostics:
- Serum: lipemia
- CBC: no overall change
- Chemistry:
  - Hyperglycemia
  - Altered liver enzymes
  - Elevations in cholesterol

Hyperglycemia: stress vs. diabetes

Urine glucose levels on at-home samples

Recheck blood glucose once patient relaxes.

Fructosamine levels

Obtain a urinalysis:
- Confirm glucosuria (differentiate from stress).
- Determine whether ketones are present.
- Identify secondary urinary tract infection.

Identify diabetic ketoacidotic patients.

Evaluate patient for primary disease that may cause diabetes secondarily (Type III):
- Adrenal axis testing (hyperadrenocorticism)
- Thyroid testing (hyperthyroidism)
- Evaluate for chronic pancreatitis:
  - Clinical chemistry
  - TLI (canine only)
  - PLI
  - Ultrasound
  - Blood folate levels

Blood Sugar

A persistent hyperglycemia (high blood sugar) is the most notable change observed. Stress can also cause elevations in blood glucose as well. Although blood levels of Glucose can vary from lab to lab, normal levels are generally as shown in Chart 7.5.

Chart 7.5

Canine	60–125 mg/dL
Feline	70–150 mg/dL

In general, the medical team should be more concerned if the patient is a diabetic whose glucose levels are the following:

Canines: Glucose > 200 mg/dL tend to be a true hyperglycemia.
Felines: Glucose < 300 mg/dL tend to be a true hyperglycemia.

If a severely stressed patient presents with questionable elevation in blood sugar, the medical team should recommend the following tests.

Check the Patient's Urine

Evidence of urine glucose can help determine whether the patient is diabetic. However, it is important to note that stressed patients (especially felines) with blood glucose above 240 mg/dL can spill some sugar into the urine, producing both a hyperglycemia and low-level glucose in the urine (**glucosuria**). The owner should bring in serial samples of urine collected **at home** to determine whether the patient has glucosuria evident in a nonstressed environment.

Repeat Blood Sugar

Repeat the blood sugar testing later during the visit once the pet has seemed to calm down.

Perform a Fructosamine Level Test

See section on fructosamine levels below.

Liver Enzymes

Mild to moderate elevations in liver enzymes (i.e., alanine transferase, aspartate transferase) can be observed with chronic diabetes. Also secondary to altered fat metabolism, blood cholesterol level elevations can be observed.

Urinalysis

The evidence of a persistent glucosuria can support the finding of hyperglycemia to confirm the diagnosis of diabetes. With concerns of Type I diabetes, the presence of urine ketones (acetone) confirming the diagnosis of ketoacidotic diabetes. Diabetic patients also can develop secondary bacterial bladder infections due to the glucosuria increasing bacterial growth of the urine. These patients will develop proteinuria, hematuria, and elevations of white blood cells, urinary crystals, and bacteria evident in the urine sediment. In many cases these urinary tract infections must also be eliminated to help chronic control of insulin need in the diabetic patient.

Fructosamine Levels

Fructosamine is a slowly metabolized blood sugar that allows the veterinarian to determine how the patient is metabolizing body sugar stores over the previous 7 to 10 days. Animals with significantly elevated fructosamine levels can suggest decreased control of insulin production and utilization. Decreased fructosamine levels can suggest that the patient may be given too much insulin, producing periods of hypoglycemia. Blood levels of fructosamine can vary from lab to lab, and reference ranges depend on the method and instrument used.

Electrolyte Physiology, Function, and Derangement

This chapter focuses on the common electrolytes monitored in an in-hospital clinical diagnostic evaluation, their function, and the conditions noted when their concentration is deranged.

Sodium

Sodium is the most abundant positively charged ion in the extracellular fluid that helps to regulate electrical potential in the body. The movement of extracellular sodium into the cell and intracellular potassium out of the cell stimulates an electrical rhythm. When the body needs to produce an electrical rhythm for muscular contraction, nerve depolarization, heart contraction, and millions of other muscular and neurological activities, sodium and potassium switch places to produce the electrical pulse necessary for the action (Figure 8.1).

The balance of sodium to potassium is critical to maintaining normal electrical potential and physiological balance. The body must maintain sodium serum levels between 140–155 mEq/ml and maintain 27 times more sodium then potassium in the extracellular fluid. The adrenal-mineralocorticoid axis (see Chapter 11) maintains the balance of sodium to potassium by producing a mineralocorticoid called aldosterone. This hormone is responsible for the reabsorption of sodium and expulsion of potassium in the distal convoluted tubules in the kidney (Figure 8.2). This hormone above all other adrenal hormones is needed for normal handling of stress and body maintenance. Without sufficient levels of this hormone, an animal can develop a life-threatening crisis.

Although blood levels of sodium can vary from lab to lab, levels generally are as shown in Chart 8.1.

Chart 8.1

| Canine | 142–150 mEq/L |
| Feline | 147–162 mEq/L |

Derangements in sodium are typically related to conditions that affect fluid

119

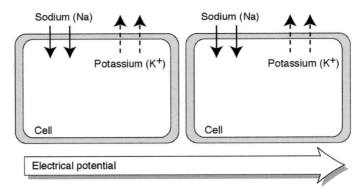

Figure 8.1. Illustration of sodium and potassium role within the cell to produce an electrical rhythm. These electrical waves maintain normal function in neurological, cardiovascular, and muscular actions.

concentration in the body. Low blood sodium levels, **hyponatremia,** is related to factors that increase solute loss in the body, most commonly seen in patients with moderate to severe vomiting and diarrhea. Hyponatremia can also be observed in association with patients with increased blood potassium, **hyperkalemia,** and in

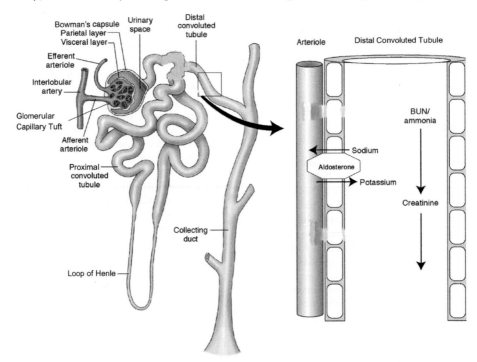

Figure 8.2. Illustration of distal tubule of a nephron of the kidney. Here the hormone aldosterone controls the reabsorbtion of sodium and expulsion of potassium from the body.

patients with decreased production of aldosterone, **hypoadrenocorticism**. Hyponatremic patients are generally lethargic and weak; however, with hyponatremia, seizures and comas have been reported.

Increased serum sodium concentration, **hypernatremia**, is observed **rarely** in patients that ingest too much salt, are given too much NaCl containing IV fluids, or have conditions where patients have increased fluid loss but maintain adequate body sodium concentrations. Hypernatremia is extremely rare; however, hypernatremic patients have increased thirst (**polydipsia**), become disoriented, and have seizures and comas.

Potassium

As discussed above, sodium and potassium are responsible for production of electrical energy in the body. However, unlike sodium, derangements in potassium are more common and can produce serious physical symptoms and potential life-threatening concerns. Although blood levels of potassium can vary from lab to lab, normal levels generally are as shown in Chart 8.2.

Chart 8.2

Canine	4.0–5.4 mEq/L
Feline	3.7–5.2 mEq/L

Hypokalemia

Hypokalemia, **potassium <2.5 mEq/L**, is associated with diseases that increase fluid loss (i.e., vomiting or diarrhea, chronic renal disease, animals on intravenous fluids) or patients that are being treated for diabetes ketoacidosis in the hospital (see Chapter 7). Common diseases associated with hypokalemia are reviewed in the following sections.

Gastrointestinal Disease

Diseases such as colitis, parvoviral infection, panleukopenia, and gastric foreign body severe can produce a profound hypokalemia (<2.5 mEq/dL) due to significant fluid losses from vomiting and diarrhea.

Renal Disease

Animals with chronic kidney disease lose the ability to concentrate urine in the renal medulla (see Chapter 5). To compensate, patients increase their fluid consumption and urine output, which increases the amount of potassium excreted.

Hospitalized Animals on IV Fluids

Hospitalized patients on intravenous fluid support that are not able to eat can develop hypokalemia due to the increased IV fluid and urinary output.

Diabetic Ketoacidotic (DKA)

DKA patients must receive regular injections (every 1–3 hours) or constant rate infusions of short-acting insulin (Humilin-N®) in order to lower blood glucose and ketone levels in the blood. As insulin increases absorption of glucose, potassium also is carried into the cell. This rapid internalization can make the patient profoundly hypokalemic.

Hypokalemia is generally not life threatening, but patients are generally weak, depressed, anorexic, and with severe conditions such as have ventroflexion of the neck (Figure 8.3).

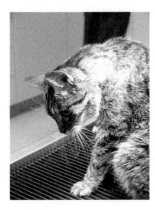

Figure 8.3.   Image of a cat unable to lift its neck due to severe hypokalemia (**ventroflexion of the neck**).

Hyperkalemia

High blood potassium level, **hyperkalemia**, is a life-threatening derangement of the body's electrolyte balance when potassium levels **exceed 5.7 mEq/mL**. Hyperkalemia can occur when patients are unable to remove potassium normally from the blood into the urine, are given too much intravenous potassium supplementation, or cannot remove urine from their body. The most common diseases that produce hyperkalemia are reviewed in the following sections.

Feline Lower Urinary Tract Disease (FLUTD) or Urinary Obstruction

Observed mostly in male felines, urinary-obstructed patients are unable to eliminate potassium from the body and can develop severe hyperkalemia.

Hypoadrenocorticism

As discussed previously, patients with decreased aldosterone production are unable to produce the excretion of potassium in the kidneys while reabsorbing sodium (see Chapter 11).

Overadministration of Potassium-Supplemented Fluids

Patients on intravenous fluids that are supplemented with potassium chloride or other potassium-containing additives can develop severe hyperkalemia when patients are given more than 0.5 mEq/kg/hr. To avoid this condition, patients should never receive boluses that also contain potassium additive.

Although rare, there are nonpathologic conditions that produce a non–life-threatening or artifactual hyperkalemia. The medical team should consider all potential causes, true and artifactual, to assure the identification of the truly hyperkalemic patient. Some causes of non–life-threatening or artifactual hyperkalemia are discussed in the following sections.

Breed Specificity

The Akita and other Japanese breeds have red blood cells with a unique Na/K pump. This pump continues to move potassium out of the cell after blood samples have been collected. These patients will have increases in their serum potassium as long as the serum and clot are in contact. Prompt separation of the serum and red cells is needed to obtain a true serum potassium concentration in these breeds.

Gastrointestinal Disease

Patients suffering from chronic gastrointestinal disease or parasitism can have significant hyponatremia and hyperkalemia. The artifactual hyperkalemia is caused by the translocation of potassium in exchange for hydrogen ions by severe metabolic acidosis. The clinical chemistry of these patients may appear very similar to the **hypoadrenocortical patient (Addisonian)**. The only way to differentiate between these two diseases is an ACTH stimulation test (see Chapter 11).

Potassium Supplementation

As discussed previously, patients that receive a bolus of potassium-rich fluids or are on high levels of oral potassium supplementation can become hyperkalemic.

Changes in Peripheral White Blood Cell and Platelet Concentrations

In rare conditions, patients with severe elevation in their white blood cell (white blood cell count >200,000) or platelet counts (>1,000,000) can have significantly increased serum potassium due to loss of potassium from these cells after the sample is obtained.

Hyperkalemia can be a life-threatening condition affecting primarily nerves and skeletal and cardiac muscle. The following are signs associated with hyperkalemia:

* Muscle fasiculations
* Pulse deficits
* Decreased mentation
* Bradycardia
* Cardiac arrhythmia
* Flaccid paralysis
* Death

Because hyperkalemia can produce serious life-threatening syndromes, the medical team must be quick and effective at evaluating blood work for the cause of the hyperkalemia as well as secondary complications that can occur. Key clinical diagnostic tests for affected patients are reviewed in the following sections.

Clinical Chemistry

The following changes in clinical chemistry should be evaluated if hyperkalemia is observed.

Hypoglycemia

Patients suffering from an acute hypoadrenocorticism (Addisonian) syndrome can become significantly hypoglycemic. Many patients with significant hypoglycemia (<60 mg/dL) may many need emergency supplementation.

Azotemia

Hypoadrenocorticism

Addisonian patients lose the ability to concentrate urine due to the inability of the renal medulla to produce a high sodium gradient. These patients develop dehydration, decreasing glomerular filtration and producing a prerenal azotemia (see Chapter 5). Unlike normal renal azotemia, the Addisonian patient will have an azotemia and dilute urine that will correct with treatment.

FLUTD or Urinary-Obstructed Patients

These patients develop postrenal azotemia due to the inability to remove urine from the body. These patients have severe azotemia, have concentrated urine (initially), and are hyperkalemic.

Sodium/Potassium Ratio (Na/K)

In the Addisonian patient, due to the inability of the kidneys to reabsorb sodium and expel potassium, the patient becomes hyponatremic and hyperkalemic. The electrolyte balance is described by the sodium/potassium ratio. **The normal ratio of sodium to potassium should always be**

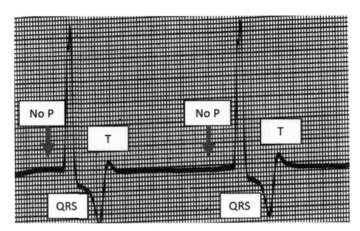

Figure 8.4.   A sample of an EKG strip with no apparent P waves. Loss of the P wave can support the diagnosis of hyperkalemia.

>25:1. When the ratio of Na/K is <23:1, Addison's disease should be suspected. There are conditions that can produce significant hyperkalemia without hyponatremia. If the Na/K ratio is low but the patient is not hyponatremic, Addison's disease is unlikely.

Electrocardiogram

Another concern that supports severe serum hyperkalemia is the **loss of the P wave (Figure 8.4) in a normal EKG strip.** Hyperkalemia can produce a small and wider P wave until it disappears entirely. If team members are concerned about severe hyperkalemia and rapid measurement of potassium concentration is not available, evaluation of the EKG strip can be used to support a diagnosis of hyperkalemia.

Chloride

Chloride is an abundant anion in the extracellular fluid. It is closely associated with sodium, and changes that produce hypo-/hypernatremia also produce similar changes in the chloride population. Although blood levels of chloride can vary from lab to lab, normal levels generally are as shown in Chart 8.3.

Chart 8.3

Canine	105–117 mEq/L
Feline	114–126 mEq/L

Similarly, physical symptoms of high chloride (hyperchloremia) and low chloride blood levels (hypochloremia) are the same as seen with changes in the sodium blood level.

Calcium

Calcium is needed by almost every cell in the body to control cellular activity, aid in muscular contraction, help heart function, and aid nerve conduction as well as other body functions. Changes in calcium concentration in the body can be observed in hormonal disease, specific types of cancer, nutritional disease, renal disease, and reproductive disease. Blood calcium exists in an inactivated protein-bound form (bound to albumin), an active ionized form, and also bound in complex with other substances. Change in blood calcium concentration can produce serious life-threatening disease. Although blood levels of Calcium can vary from lab to lab, normal levels generally are as shown in Chart 8.4.

Chart 8.4

Canine	9.2–11.2 mg/dL
Feline	7.2–11.4 mg/dL

Hypocalcemia

Low blood calcium, hypocalcemia, is rarely seen in disease conditions of the dog and cat. Most commonly, patients that are hypoalbuminemic from other causes (e.g., chronic bleeding and liver, renal or intestinal disease), will have an artifactual hypocalcemia. This is due to the fact that a large percentage of blood calcium is complexed with albumin; therefore, a decreased albumin level can produce a hypocalcemia state. Pathologic hypocalcemia is most commonly associated with those conditions reviewed in the following sections.

Eclampsia, Postparturient Hypocalcemia

Eclampsia is a serious condition of the pregnant dog shortly after pregnancy due to increased demands of blood calcium secondary to lactation. Once lactation begins, calcium levels fall rapidly and the patient cannot compensate, and the muscular, cardiac, and neurologic systems are severely affected. The disease is more common in small breed dogs, more predominantly during the first litter, and lactating females are usually affected within the first 2 weeks after birth. It is important to note that eclamptic patients can also be severely hypoglycemic. Signs occur acutely and the owners will usually report the following clinical signs:

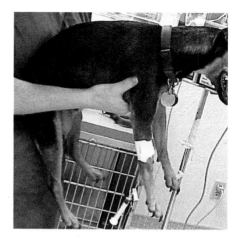

Figure 8.5. Image of a female dog with eclampsia. Hypocalcemia prevents normal muscle contraction, so the patients often appear rigid with a sawhorselike stance and muscle fasiculations.

- Restlessness
- Nervousness
- Whining
- Muscular tremors
- Slow heart rate (**bradycardia**)
- Walking stiffly (Figure 8.5)
- Seizurelike activity
- Rapid respiratory rates
- Convulsions
- High body temperature (secondary to muscular spasms)

Acute/Chronic Renal Failure

Patients with acute/chronic renal failure can develop hypocalcemia.

Ethylene Glycol Intoxication

Antifreeze intoxication can also produce hypocalcemia.

Hypercalcemia

High blood levels of calcium, hypercalcemia, is a more serious disease concern potentially affecting renal, gastrointestinal, cardiac, and other soft tissues of the body. Prolonged hypercalcemia can produce abnormal calcification of the body, leading to kidney failure, bladder stone formation (calcium oxalate), altered gastrointestinal function, abnormal contractility, and hypertension. Hypercalcemia is produced from specific types of cancer (**hypercalcemia of malignancy—e.g., lymphoma, leukemia, anal gland adenocarcinoma**), overproduction of a calcium-releasing hormone—**parathyroid hormone (PTH)**, acute renal failure, types of rat poison ingestion, hypoadrenocorticism, and specific infectious diseases (e.g., blastomycosis). Typically, physical signs observed are based the underlying disease producing the hypercalcemia. **Although not an emergency finding, team members identifying a hypercalcemic patient should discuss their concerns with the veterinarian.**

secondary to disease conditions. However, similar to potassium, significant hypophosphotemia can result from acid/base imbalance and aggressive insulin therapy when treating a diabetic ketoacidotic animal. Patients on prolonged short-acting insulin therapy (>24 hours) can develop a significant hypophosphotemia, and **serum phosphorus levels <1.0 mg/dL can result in a hemolytic crisis.** Signs associated with decreased phosphorus concentration include the following:

- Pale MM
- Rapid respiratory and cardiac rates
- Red urine and serum
- Spherocyte formation (Figure 8.6)
- Weakness
- Depression

Phosphorus

Similar to calcium, phosphorus is a mineral integral to many cell functions including bone formation, energy metabolism, muscle contraction, and acid/base balance. Phosphorus is absorbed in the diet and stored with calcium in a complex architecture that gives bone its strength. Phosphorus is also a key element needed for energy production in the cell. Although blood levels of phosphorus can vary from lab to lab, normal levels generally are as shown in Chart 8.5.

Chart 8.5

Canine	2.3–5.5 mg/dL
Feline	3.0–7.0 mg/dL

Hypophosphotemia

Decreased phosphorus concentration hypophosphotemia is not generally produced

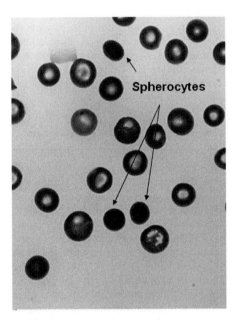

Figure 8.6. Concerns of a hemolytic anemia produced by hypophosphotemia produces spherocytes in the blood film.

Table 8.1. Electrolyte abnormalities, their causes, and their secondary concerns.

Element	Normal Finding	Presence of Abnormality Suggests
Sodium	Canine: 142–150 mEq/L Feline: 147–162 mEq/L	**Hyponatremia:** Associated with loss of solute from vomiting and diarrhea and hypoadrenocorticism. **Evaluate potassium levels.** **Hypernatremia:** Associated with increased intake and loss of large quantities of fluids.
Potassium	Canine: 4.0–5.4 mEq/L Feline: 3.7–5.2 mEq/L	**Hypokalemia:** Associated with chronic gastrointestinal loss (vomiting/diarrhea), chronic renal disease, and long-term IV fluid therapy. Severe hypokalemia can be associated with treatment of the DKA patient. **Hyperkalemia:** • **Artifactual hyperkalemia** can be associated with specific breeds (Japanese canine breeds), chronic intestinal/parasitic disease, and severe abnormalities in white blood cell count and platelet count. • **Disease:** Associated with hypoadrenocorticism and urinary obstruction. **Evaluate sodium level.**
Chloride	Canine: 105–117 mEq/L Feline: 114–126 mEq/L	**Hypochloremia:** Closely associated with causes of hyponatremia and loss of solute. **Hyperchloremia:** Closely associated with hypernatremia and increased intake and loss of large quantities of fluids.
Calcium	Canine: 9.2–11.2 mg/dL Feline: 7.2–11.4 mg/dL	**Hypocalcemia:** Associated with eclampsia, acute/chronic renal failure, and ethylene glycol intoxication. **Hypercalcemia:** Associated with specific types of cancers, acute renal failure, overproduction of parathyroid hormone, hypoadrenocorticism, specific rodenticides, and specific types of infection.
Phosphorus	Canine: 2.3–5.5 mg/dL Feline: 3.0–7.0 mg/dL	**Hypophosphotemia:** Associated with the treatment of the DKA patient. If levels are <1.0 mg/dL, hypophosphotemia can produce a hemolytic anemia. **Hyperphosphotemia:** Associated with decreased excretion of phosphorus from the kidneys secondary to renal disease and failure. Can be also associated with diseases that produce severe prerenal and postrenal azotemia (see Chapter 5).

Hyperphosphotemia

Increased levels of serum phosphorus (hyperphosphotemia) are most commonly associated with decreased excretion of phosphorus from the kidneys secondary to renal disease and failure. However, hyperphosphotemia can also be associated with diseases that produce severe prerenal and postrenal azotemia (see Chapter 5). Physical symptoms of hyperphosphotemia are dependent on the underlying disease causing the aberration (Table 8.1).

Components of the Urinalysis

The urinalysis is one of the most important tests available for evaluating an ill patient, as well as for monitoring well patients. The test is inexpensive, but it requires a skilled technician. It is highly recommended that this test is done in-house because fresh urine that is evaluated within 2–4 hours of collection will provide the most valid findings. There are many parameters on the chemistry profile that cannot be interpreted without a urinalysis. The evaluation of renal function values, protein concentration, and metabolic function requires information that is provided in the urinalysis. The complete urinalysis is the evaluation of the physical (color, clarity, and specific gravity), chemical, and formed element characteristics of urine.

Obtaining the Sample

Sampling technique has a significant effect on the results of the urinalysis and their interpretation. A sterile container should be used when obtaining a urine sample if a urine culture is anticipated. **The preferred collection methods are cystocentesis and catheterization.** Less useful methods are free-catch and bladder expression. Secretions from the lower urinary tract affect both free catch and bladder expression. If the only way to obtain a sample is with a free catch, a midstream urine catch is preferred to decrease contamination. Regardless, if the examination of the urine reveals abnormal findings such as bacteria or increased protein, a cystocentesis or catheterized sample must be obtained to confirm that the abnormalities are related to disease in the kidneys or urinary bladder. An additional problem with bladder expression is the small but real possibility of a ruptured bladder if excessive pressure is used or the bladder wall is compromised.

The timing of a urinalysis can be important in obtaining the most information from a urine collection. **A first morning sample (obtained just after the patient is taken out of its cage in the morning) will provide the best evaluation of concentrating ability.** It is also the best sample to evaluate for formed elements such as casts. The urinalysis should be done as soon as possible after obtaining the sample. Cellular element and crystals can deteriorate, making it difficult to recognize these structures correctly. In addition, crystals may dissolve or form over time. Chemical parameters can also change as urine sits, especially at room temperature. If the urinalysis must be postponed, **the urine can be refrigerated for no longer than 6 hours.** If the sample is refrigerated, it must be allowed to return to room temperature before the chemical analysis is done. Several of the indicator pads on the reagent strip are enzyme-based reactions. The speed of enzymatic reactions decreases as temperature decreases; therefore, the timing for reading the reaction will not be valid unless the urine is at room temperature.

A standard operating procedure (SOP), as discussed in Chapter 1, is important to ensure that the urinalysis results are obtained and reported in a uniform manner. For quality assurance, the following information should be recorded on a urinalysis record for each sample: when the sample was obtained, how the sample was obtained, any medication given prior to the urinalysis, and when the urinalysis was performed. A legible label containing the patient's name, owner and hospital ID number should be placed on the container (not the lid) at the time of collection.

There are controls available for urinalysis. These are expensive and are not routinely used. For most cases, if the reagent strips are handled and stored properly and not used passed their expiration date, controls do not need to be performed. There are reagents that can be used to test the laboratory technician's sediment evaluation skills. These controls are helpful for in-house quality assurance programs and for technician training.

The common sources of error in urinalysis are primarily preanalytical (inappropriate collection) and analytical. The most common preanalytical error is contamination of the urine during sample collection. The temptation to analyze urine that has been collected from any surface (however clean it is thought to be) should be avoided if at all possible. Unfortunately, it is difficult to prevent a patient from evacuating its bladder before a cystocentesis or catheterization procedure. If the only sample that can be obtained is from the surface of the examination table, the results must be provided with major disclaimers on the interpretation of certain elements of the urinalysis. Cleaning solvents can alter the chemical reactions on the reagent pads; therefore, a chemical evaluation should not be reported. The presence of bacteria cannot be interpreted, because bacteria from the surface will contaminate the sample. The specific gravity will usually not be altered and crystals or formed elements such as erythrocytes, leukocytes, and casts can still be reported.

The following are the most common analytical errors:

1. Delay in performing urinalysis without refrigeration
2. Failure to mix the sample prior to aliquoting
3. Failure to adequately resuspend the sample
4. Failure to follow the standard operating procedure with specific adherence to the volume of aliquot evaluated, centrifuge speed and time, and number of high power fields evaluated.

Performing the Analysis

A routine urinalysis includes the following steps:

1. Collect urine in a sterile container or syringe.

2. Mix the urine gently and place a standard volume (5 or 10 mL) of the urine in a conical centrifuge tube.
3. Record color and clarity and perform the chemical analysis.
4. Centrifuge for 3–5 min at 1000–2000 rpm (~100 G).
5. Record volume of sediment using the graduations on the conical tube.
6. Pour off the **supernatant** (leave a standard volume of supernatant to resuspend the sediment, 0.3–0.5 ml).
7. Place a drop of the resuspended sediment **pellet** on a glass slide and place a coverslip over the drop.

Gross Evaluation

Normal urine is clear and light to dark yellow in color. Urine can have a rainbow of colors, however; diet, disease, and drugs can alter the color of urine. The most common abnormal colors seen in urine are red/orange, black/brown, and green. When methylene blue was being used as a urine acidifier, it caused the urine to be bluish. Black or brown discoloration of the urine is seen with methemoglobin and nitrites. Green discoloration is seen when bilirubin is present and allowed to break down over time. The most common color changes seen in veterinary samples are red, red-brown, red-orange, and orange. These colors all relate to the presence of erythrocytes or heme pigments in the urine (**hemoglobin, myoglobin, porphyrin**).

Hematuria is indicated when the urine is red and turbid (cloudy). When a hematuric urine sample is spun, the erythrocytes will pellet at the bottom of the tube, and the supernatant will be clear or translucent. **Hemoglobinuria and myoglobinuria** is indicated when the urine is red and translucent. When **hemoglobinuric** or **myoglobinuric** urine is spun down, the color remains in the supernatant and no erythrocyte pellet will form. Although there are diagnostic tests that can be performed on urine to differentiate myoglobin from hemoglobin, the easiest way is to evaluate a concurrent blood serum sample. Hemoglobinuric patients will also be **hemoglobinemic**. Myoglobinuric patients will have clear serum. Myoglobin is cleared from the serum by the kidney very rapidly, but it takes much longer to clear hemoglobin.

Urine Specific Gravity

The specific gravity of urine depends on the number and type of solutes (soluble particles) in the urine. The specific gravity is measured using a refractometer, often the same one that is used to measure total protein in body cavity fluids and plasma. The specific gravity of distilled water is 1.000. Distilled water can be used to check the calibration of the **refractometer**. Large amounts of protein and glucose can increase the specific gravity of a urine sample. There are refractometers made specifically for veterinary samples. These instruments have one scale for dogs and large animal species that goes to up to 1.045 and another scale for cats that goes up to 1.060. Any urine sample with specific gravity that goes beyond the scale should be recorded as greater than the highest reading on the appropriate scale (>1.045 or >1.060). There is no reference range for urine specific gravity in the normal patient. The specific gravity will vary depending on the hydration status. In general, the expected USG in a patient that is dehydrated but has normal renal function should be as shown in Chart 9.1.

Chart 9.1

Canine	USG >1.030
Feline	USG >1.035

Chemical Evaluation

Chemical analysis of the urine can be performed on the supernatant of the centrifuged sample or on uncentrifuged urine. The primary reason for performing the analysis on uncentrifuged urine is the fact that centrifugation will clear the blood cells from the urine and may cause a false negative reading on the blood reagent pad. However, erythrocytes will be seen on the microscopic evaluation if present in numbers too small to see grossly. The advantage of performing the analysis on centrifuged samples is to clear the urine of particulates that may interfere with interpretation of the reagent pad changes. Chemical analysis of the urine must be done when the urine is at room temperature. When done on cold urine from the refrigerator, many of the reagent pads will be falsely negative or less positive.

The package insert for the reagent strip usually has a recommended procedure to follow. It will also have a list of substances that may interfere with the reagent reactions if they are present in the urine. It is important to ensure that the cross-contamination of the individual reagent pads does not occur. The urine should be aliquoted into the conical centrifuge tube before the chemical analysis is done. It is best to tilt the tube toward the horizontal plane, immerse the reagent test strip, and quickly remove it, drawing the strip across the edge of the tube into a horizontal position. Do not allow urine to run from one pad to the next. Alternatively, urine can be drawn into a small syringe and aliquots placed directly on each test pad.

Each pad has a specific incubation time that must be followed before the color of the pad can be interpreted. It is very helpful to review the times for each test in the package insert before performing the test to know what order and time they should be read. As indicated previously, there are artifacts that can interfere with interpretation of the color change on the reagent pads.

The package insert should list confounding factors for each individual test. Some of the most common artifacts are seen with the tests reviewed in the following sections.

Glucose

The glucose reagent pad is enzyme dependent; therefore, it is sensitive to temperature. Ascorbic acid will cause a false negative. Some glucose reagent pads will have decreased activity in urine with a low (<1.005) specific gravity. Contamination of the urine sample with cleaning agents can cause a false positive. Strict adherence to the expiration date is necessary, and the enzyme activity will decrease rapidly after the expiration date.

Ketones

The ketone reaction on the reagent pad will detect only one of the ketoacids that may be in the urine. Therefore, a negative reaction does not entirely rule out ketonuria. The reaction is highly sensitive to moisture, heat, and light, so it is important to tightly replace the lid on the reagent strip bottle. False positive ketone reactions can be seen with administration of captopril, D-penicillamine, tiopronin, and cystine.

Conjugated Bilirubin

Conjugated bilirubin, the form of bilirubin excreted in the urine, can be quickly degraded to biliverdin or unconjugated bilirubin, both of which do not react with the reagent pad. Dark-colored urine will make interpretation of the bilirubin reaction difficult. Ascorbic acid in the urine can result in a false negative result in some test strips.

Blood

The test pad for blood will react with erythrocytes, hemoglobin, and myoglobin. Some test strips can differentiate low numbers of intact erythrocytes from hemoglobin and myoglobin because intact red cells will cause a stippled appearance rather than a solid color change. However, a large number of intact erythrocytes will result in a solid color change, the same as hemoglobin or myoglobin.

Protein

For most reagent strips, the protein pad detects albumin. Highly alkaline urine can result in a false positive reaction in some test strips. The reaction of the protein pad should be interpreted in concert with the urine specific gravity. A 1+ urine protein in a urine sample with 1.010 specific gravity is more significant than a 1+ finding in a sample with 1.040 specific gravity.

Nonuseful Reagent Pads

There are reagent strips that include specific gravity, nitrate, and leukocyte reactions. None of these reactions are useful in the veterinary patient. Urobilinogen is sometime present on reagent strips as well. This reaction, for the most part, is not useful. It is very insensitive because urobilinogen is very unstable. Some sulfa-based antibiotics will cause false positive reactions. The pH of the urine can have a great effect on the reaction. Highly alkaline urine will increase the reaction, and acid urine can decrease the reaction. When choosing a reagent test strip for use in the clinic, consider ones that do not have these tests. It is not worth paying for tests that are of little use.

Sediment Examination

Examination of urine sediment can be done with or without sediment stain. Unstained specimens have fewer artifacts, but they are more difficult for some individuals to evaluate. Using stain adds to the cost of the

procedure and is considered a "crutch" by many laboratory microscopists. The sediment (stained or unstained) is dropped onto a glass slide and a uniform coverslip is placed over the urine drop. The size of the coverslip is not significant, other than the fact that the large coverslip allows more area for evaluation. The slide is placed on the microscope stage and the light is adjusted by closing the iris diaphragm or lowering the stage just as one would do when counting white blood cells in a hemocytometer.

The sediment examination is performed by scanning the urine on low power (10× objective) to identify large formed elements such as epithelial cells and casts of renal tubules. The entire coverslip is scanned at low power and the average number of formed elements per low power field is recorded (i.e., 1–2 squamous cells/**low power field [lpf]**). Following the low power scan, a consistent predetermined number of high power fields (40× objectives) are evaluated. At this power, the type of cells in the urine can be better identified and recorded as cells/**high power field (hpf)**. The cellular elements that can be seen in urine include squamous cells, transitional cells, white blood cells, and erythrocytes. Other formed elements, bacteria, fungi, and crystals are identified and reported at few, moderate, or many. The type of crystal is identified and the morphology of any microorganism is recorded.

The most difficult part of the urinalysis for most technicians is evaluation of the sediment. Confidence and competence requires practice. Making urinalysis a routine test for all sick patients and part of a wellness examination will allow constant honing of microscopy skills by the technician. The formed elements in the urine sediment that should be easily identified by any technician doing a urinalysis include erythrocytes, white blood cells, epithelial cells (squamous and transitional), casts, crystals, and bacteria.

Erythrocytes

Erythrocytes are the smallest of the cellular elements. They can be found in small numbers in normal samples (0–3/HPF), especially in cystocentesis samples. They are small round biconcave disks with slight reddish to greenish tinge. If the urine has a high specific gravity, the red cells may be crenated. In urine with a low specific gravity, the erythrocytes may lyse and faint ghost membranes may be seen.

Erythrocytes are most easily confused with white blood cells and fat droplets. Cat urine tends to have a significant number of fat droplets. White blood cells are larger and have a granular pattern. They will appear lighter than the erythrocyte. Fat droplets vary in size and usually collect just under the coverslip in a plane above the erythrocytes. Focusing up and down will show the different planes for these two elements.

White Blood Cells

White blood cells can also be found in normal urine in low numbers (0–2/HPF). Leukocytes are larger than erythrocytes and have a granular appearance (they seem to glitter as you focus up and down). In some cases, you will see the segmented nucleus of the neutrophil.

Epithelial Cells

Epithelial cells are larger than erythrocytes and leukocytes. Squamous epithelial cells are found in higher numbers in free catch samples. They are the largest cells found in urine sediment. They have abundant cytoplasm, small round nuclei, and angular edges.

Transitional cells (urothelial cells) vary considerably in size, have rounded edges, and have variable amounts of cytoplasm. Their nucleus is round. This cell type can be quite reactive when there is an inflammatory process present in the urinary bladder. If there is suspicion of transitional cell neoplasia, a urine sample can be sent in for further evaluation by a cytopathologist.

Microorganisms

Bacteria and artifacts that can imitate bacteria cause the greatest confusion on a urinalysis. Both rods and coccoid bacteria can be seen in the urine of patients with a septic process of the urinary tract. The most common type of bacteria seen in urinary infections is rod-shaped and motile. As a result, on examination of the sediment when these bacteria are present, the microscopist should see small rod-shaped organisms with progressive movement.

When coccoid bacteria are seen, it is important to see them in chains or organized clusters. Most coccoid bacteria are nonmotile, so forward motion will not be seen. Brownian motion is random motion by particles suspended in a liquid. Many urine samples have small particulate matter such as very small crystals or amorphous debris that is round and about the size of coccoid bacteria. When suspended in the urine, they will vacillate in place, but they will not show progressive forward motion. **In most cases, when bacteria are present, leukocytes will be present as well.** If you identify bacteria and there isn't an inflammatory response indicated by the presence of **pyuria** (neutrophils in the urine), the bacteria are likely contaminants. The exception to this rule is when an animal is immunosuppressed, receiving corticosteroids, or has Cushing's disease.

Fungi are less common in urine samples than bacteria. Yeast is the most common fungal elements seen; however, fungi that form hyphie or mycelia can be found in some cases. Yeast are larger than bacteria and are occasionally confused with erythrocytes. With close examination, budding yeast can usually be found. The budding yeast body can have a thin or broad base, and this characteristic can be helpful in identification of possible species of yeast. Yeast can be contaminates from the lower urinary tract when a free-catch sample is evaluated.

There are very few parasites that are found in the urinary tract. Though rare, ova of the bladder worm, *Capillaria pica*, or *Capillaria felis* can be found in urine from dogs and cats.

Urinary Casts

Casts are formed elements that are literally "casts" of the tubules in which they form. Casts can be cellular (erythrocytes, leukocytes, or renal tubular cells), granular (coarse, fine), hyaline (protein), or waxy.

Hyaline casts are clear, colorless, and refractile. They have parallel sides and consist of protein.

Granular casts are the most common casts seen in the urine. They consist of degenerate cellular debris. Granular casts often have a yellow/brown hue.

Cellular casts consist of recognizable cells. They can be composed of leukocytes, renal tubular epithelial cells, and erythrocytes. Red cell casts will have the same red to greenish hue seen in the free erythrocytes in urine. **Cellular casts are not common.** Their presence in urine is highly significant. White blood cell casts are seen in pyonephritis and indicate significant inflammation within the renal tubules. Red cell casts confirm hemorrhage into the renal tubules. Epithelial cell casts indicate acute sloughing of the renal tubular epithelial cells.

Waxy casts indicate chronic renal disease with low glomerular filtration rate (low flow of urine through the renal tubular system). They are the largest casts found in urine. They are clear, colorless, and refractile with "cracks" at the edge. They are formed from the lipid present in degenerate cell membranes.

Fatty casts are most common in the cat. The cat has higher lipid content in its renal tubular epithelial cells. Fatty casts have large numbers of distinct round refractile bodies embedded in a protein background. They are often accompanied by a large number of lipid droplets in the background.

Additional formed elements that can be seen in the urine include spermatozoa, parasites, and plant spores.

Urinary Crystals

There are numerous crystals that can be seen in urine samples. The type and number of each crystal should be reported.

Triple phosphate or struvite crystals are the most common crystal seen in companion animal urine. These crystals are described as "coffin lids." They are elongate with sharp edges and are usually found in slightly acidic urine. They are commonly found in urine from animals with no evidence of urinary tract disease.

Ammonium biurate crystals are a common finding in urine samples. They are brown, round, and have irregularly spaced spikes on their surface. Their presence in urine is indicative of high serum ammonia levels and is commonly associated with dogs that have a portosystemic venous shunt. However, they can be seen with severe primary hepatic disease and in the dalmatian dog.

Calcium oxalate crystals have become more common in companion animal species due to dietary changes. In an attempt to limit the formation of struvite uroliths (triple phosphate stones in the urinary system), diets have been modified to alter the acidity of the urine to make it less compatible with formation of triple phosphate stones. As a result, calcium oxalate stones have become more common. There are two forms of calcium oxalate crystals: dihydrate calcium oxalate and monohydrate calcium oxalate. It is very important to report

Table 9.1.   Elements of urine and their meanings.

Urinary Element	Normal Finding	Presence of Abnormality Suggests
Urine specific gravity	Canine >1.030 Feline >1.035	Decreased urine specific gravity can suggest the kidneys' inability to concentrate urine. This can occur simply due to increased fluid intake (oral, IV fluids) or be secondary to renal or hormonal diseases.
Urine glucose (glucosuria)	Negative	**Artifact:** Decreased USG <1.005 can hide glucosuria on the reagent strip (false negative). Contamination of the urine may produce a false positive. **Disease:** True glucosuria suggests diabetes mellitus or stress-associated hyperglycemia and glucosuria (see Chapter 7).
Urine ketones (ketonuria)	Negative	**Artifact:** Test checks for only one kind of ketone, so a negative does not always rule out ketonuria. False positive ketone reactions can be seen with administration of captopril, D-penicillamine, Tiopronin, and cystine. **Disease:** A true ketonuria with glucosuria suggests that the patient is suffering from diabetic ketoacidosis (see Chapter 7).
Conjugated bilirubin (bilirubinuria)	Negative	**Artifact:** Can show false negatives due to the presence of ascorbic acid. **Disease:** Can support evidence of liver disease, IMHA, or gallbladder obstruction in the patient.
Blood (hematuria)	Negative	**Artifact:** Test can show positive for blood, hemoglobin, or myoglobin. Diseases that cause erythrocyte destruction (e.g., IMHA) or muscle degeneration or necrosis can cause increased release of hemoglobin or myoglobin and make this test falsely positive. To help confirm the diagnosis of hematuria, the urine supernatant should be evaluated after the urine is spun. Patients with true hematuria will have a clear supernatant because the cells have been condensed into the pellet. **Disease:** Hematuria suggests that disease causes bleeding into the urinary bladder—e.g., urinary tract infections, coagulopathies, urinary stones (urolithiasis), or bladder/renal tumors.
Protein (proteinuria)	Canine: negative to trace Feline: negative	**Artifact:** Artifactual proteinuria can occur if urine pH is alkaline (>7.5). **Disease:** The presence of urine protein (especially in dilute urine) can suggest evidence of urinary tract disease or renal disease with glomerular damage.
Sediment—white blood cells	(<0–2 WBC hpf)	Evidence of increased white blood cells supports the presence of infection or inflammation within the urinary tract. Increased white blood cells are most commonly observed with urinary tract infections.

Table 9.1.   (Continued)

Urinary Element	Normal Finding	Presence of Abnormality Suggests
Sediment—erythrocytes	(<0–3 WBC hpf)	Evidence of increased erythrocytes supports the presence of bleeding within the kidney or bladder, suggesting urinary tract infections, urinary stones, or bladder or renal tumors.
Sediment—epithelial cells	(<1–2/lpf)	Increased evidence of epithelial cells can suggest the presence of some types of bladder cancer. When noted, the urinary sample should be sent to the lab for cytological evaluation.
Sediment—bacteria or fungus	None	True bacterial or fungal elements in the urine supports renal or urinary tract infection. If these elements are noted, the type of microorganism should be documented. The presence of white blood cells helps to further confirm that an infection is evident.
Casts—hyaline	Negative	Increased loss of protein in the urine.
Casts—granular	Negative	Sloughing of the renal tubular epithelial cells.
Casts—cellular	Negative	**Uncommon**. Their presence suggests serious renal disease, and its cause is dependent on the type of cell found. Erythrocyte casts suggest renal hemorrhage, whereas white blood cell casts suggest renal inflammation.
Casts—waxy	Negative	If evident, they can suggest chronic renal tubular damage secondary to chronic kidney disease.
Casts—fatty	Negative	Not significant
Crystals—triple phosphate	Negative	**Artifact:** Can precipitate out in samples that sit for too long at room temperature. **Disease:** Suggestive of crystallization of magnesium, phosphorus, and ammonia out of dietary elements in urine with an alkaline pH; usually not significant.
Crystals—calcium oxalate	Negative	**Artifact:** Can precipitate out in samples that sit for too long at room temperature. **Disease:** Suggestive of crystallization of calcium and oxalate out of dietary elements in urine with an acidic pH; usually not significant
Crystals—monohydrate calcium oxalate	Negative	These crystals are evident with ethylene glycol intoxication (antifreeze) within the first 8 hours of ingestion.
Crystals—bilirubin	Negative	Normal findings in concentrated urine in dogs; can suggest diseases that produce hyperbilirubinemia (e.g., liver disease, gallbladder obstruction, or IMHA).
Crystals—ammonium biurate crystals	Negative	Evident in patients with liver dysfunction and in dalmatians.

each specific type. Dihydrate calcium ox-alate crystals are common in the urine of dogs and cats with no evidence of renal or urinary tract disease. The dihydrate crystal is square with a refractile cross in the center. The monohydrate form is elongate with a blunt point on each end that causes it to resemble a picket fence post. The monohy-drate form is highly associated with ethy-lene glycol (antifreeze) poisoning.

Bilirubin crystals are more common in the dog than the cat. They are elongate thin yellow/brown needles that are often gath-ered into a cluster that resembles a wheat bundle. When found in the cat, they are highly associated with hyperbilirubinemia. They are considered normal findings in con-centrated urine in the dog.

Cystine crystals are rarely seen. They are indicative of a hereditary metabolic defect and cystinuria. They are perfect six-sided flat plates (hexagons).

Tests for Evaluating Changes in Glomerular Filtration

As discussed in Chapter 5, detection of pro-teinuria can be a key diagnostic test in de-termining early renal disease prior to the patient developing azotemia and physical symptoms. If renal disease is detected early, these patients can be treated to slow the pro-gression of the disease. The following sec-tions review clinical diagnostics that help evaluate these changes

Microlevels of Albumin in the Urine

An in-clinic test for very small amounts of albumin (microprotein) is available. This test can be used in detecting early re-nal disease and monitoring response to treatment.

Protein/Creatinine Ratio

This ratio is a better quantitation of pro-tein loss than the semiquantitative measure-ment of the reagent pad. It closely corre-lates with the urine protein measurement that requires collection of urine over a full 24 hours.

Endocrine Tests

The urine cortisol/creatinine ratio, per-formed in a reference laboratory, is used as a screening test for hyperadrenocorti-cism (Cushing's disease; see Chapter 11). Cortisol is a hormone that is produced by the adrenal glands to help maintain blood glucose in times of stress. In nor-mal patients, very small amounts of cor-tisol are released in the urine. In patients with increased release of cortisol secondary to Cushing's disease or other chronic dis-eases, large amounts of cortisol may be excreted in the urine. If the ratio of cor-tisol to creatinine is low, Cushing's dis-ease is highly unlikely, lowering the clinical concern. If the ratio is elevated, additional confirmatory testing for Cushing's disease (low-dose dexamethazone test or ACTH stimulation test) must be done. In general, patients with chronic diseases are stressed and will have a high cortisol/creatinine ratio (Table 9.1).

Evaluating the Urinalysis with Disease Conditions

Urinalysis is an essential component of the initial evaluation of an ill patient and the wellness exam of healthy animals (see Algorithm 10.1). Findings in the urinalysis can assist in evaluation of liver function, renal function, endocrine function, and acid-base status. Understanding how disease affects the composition of urine enables the veterinary technician to anticipate the request of additional testing by the veterinarian.

Each component of the urinalysis provides valuable information. Both abnormal and normal urinalysis findings are important in interpretation of additional diagnostic tests. Examination of the chemical composition of the urine and the sediment are required to realize the full benefit of a urinalysis. Although it is tempting to omit the sediment examination in samples with a normal chemical composition evaluated by the reagent pads, the sediment from all samples should be examined. Information concerning the urinalysis findings in several organ systems is found in several chapters within this text. This chapter pulls that in-formation together to provide an overview of urinalysis findings in disease.

Urine Specific Gravity

The specific gravity of urine is one of the most important values obtained in a urinalysis. The volume necessary to obtain a specific gravity is very small (~100 μL). It is an essential value for determination of the underlying cause of azotemia in an ill patient. As discussed in Chapter 5, there are three types of azotemia: prerenal (dehydration), renal, and postrenal (obstruction). Urine specific gravity is essential for differentiating prerenal from renal azotemia. The dehydrated azotemic patient will have a high urine specific gravity (>1.035 in the dog, >1.045 in the cat). If the urine specific gravity is less than expected for dehydration, there is an underlying defect in urine concentration that may be due to primary renal disease (loss of renal tubular function)

Algorithm 10.1. Evaluating urine color, turbidity, and specific gravity.

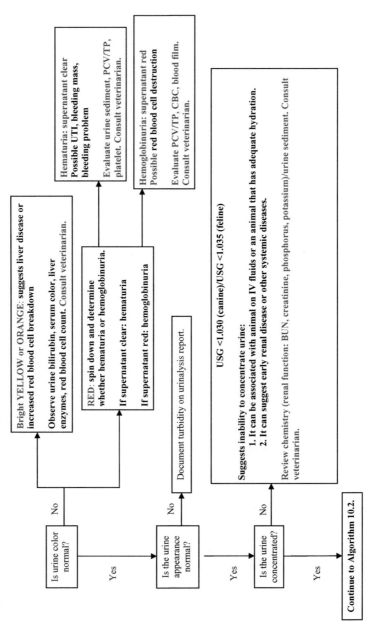

Table 10.1. Common causes of decreased urine-concentrating ability.

Loss of response to antidiuretic hormone	Glucocorticoids Hypercalcemia Hypokalemia
Osmotic diuresis	Hyperglycemia Loss of sodium into urine
Primary renal disease	Loss of renal tubule function

or secondary disease that is causing inhibition of renal tubular function. Table 10.1 lists diseases that inhibit the kidney's ability to concentrate urine and their underlying pathogenic mechanism.

Normal renal tubular function is necessary to both concentrate and dilute urine. Therefore, an azotemic animal that has a very low specific gravity (<1.005) has normal renal tubular function with an underlying disease that is not allowing normal response to **antidiuretic hormone (ADH)**, the hormone that allows the renal collecting ducts to reabsorb water from the urine as it flows through the medulla.

Primary (central) diabetes insipidus, a relatively rare disease, is a genetic disease that has been found in several breeds of dog (Great Dane, Portuguese Water Dog, Rottweiler, Standard Poodle, West Highland White Terrier, Soft-coated Wheaten Terrier, Bearded Collie, Leonberger, and Nova Scotia Duck Tolling Retriever). Primary diabetes insipidus is the lack of antidiuretic hormone. Secondary Diabetes insipidus occurs when the renal collecting ducts do not respond to ADH. In both cases, the urine specific gravity is less than 1.005. Figure 10.1 illustrates the effects of ADH and how it increases water reabsorption in the collecting ducts.

In addition to disease processes, it is important to remember that intravenous fluid and diuretic therapy will also inhibit renal concentrating ability. In an azotemic pa-

tient with a history of fluid therapy or administration of a diuretic, the urine specific gravity cannot be used to differentiate prerenal from renal azotemia. In these cases, response to appropriate therapy will determine whether the patient has adequate renal function.

Chemical Evaluation

The chemical evaluation of urine can provide information essential to disease diagnosis and interpretation of the CBC and chemistry profile (Algorithm 10.2). The chemical reagent pads on urine reagent strips provide a semiquantitative value for each substance being tested. It is important to remember that there is a degree of subjective analysis when reading the reagents pad reactions. In some cases, a more accurate evaluation may be necessary, as is often needed when determining the significance of proteinuria.

Glucosuria

Glucose is filtered out of the blood as it passes through the glomerulus and must be reabsorbed by the proximal convoluted tubules. In the normal dog and cat, all of the glucose filtered can be reabsorbed as long as the renal tubular epithelial cells are healthy and the amount of glucose filtered out does not exceed the ability of the epithelial cells to reabsorb glucose. The proximal convoluted tubular epithelial cells have specific membrane transport pumps that are responsible for moving glucose from the urine back into the serum. The renal glucose threshold is the serum glucose concentration over which the renal tubules transport pumps cannot reabsorb all of the glucose that is filtered into the urine. The renal glucose threshold is 180 mg/dL for the dog and 240 mg/dL for the cat. If the patient is

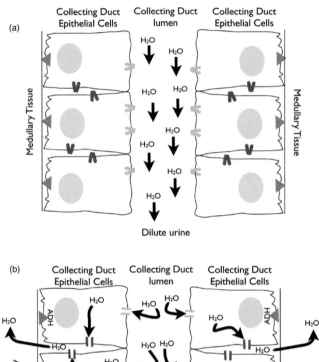

Figure 10.1. (a) The water channels are closed if there is no ADH present on the ADH receptors at the basal membrane of the renal tubule cell. Water is not reabsorbed and dilute urine is formed. (b) When ADH attaches to the ADH receptor, it changes conformation and signals the cell to open the water channels to allow water to enter the epithelial cell at the luminal surface of the cells and flow into the interstitial tissue, forming concentrated urine.

hyperglycemic with serum glucose greater than 180 mg/dL in the dog and 240 mg/dL in the cat, the patient will have glucosuria.

Glucosuria can occur when a patient's serum glucose is less than the renal glucose threshold if there is a defect in the ability of the renal tubule epithelial cells to reabsorb glucose or if there was transient hyperglycemia. There are genetic diseases that result in abnormal glucose transport pumps that cannot reabsorb glucose adequately: **Fanconi Syndrome**, seen most commonly in the basenji is one example. These patients will have normal blood glucose

Algorithm 10.2. Evaluating urine chemistry—key factors.

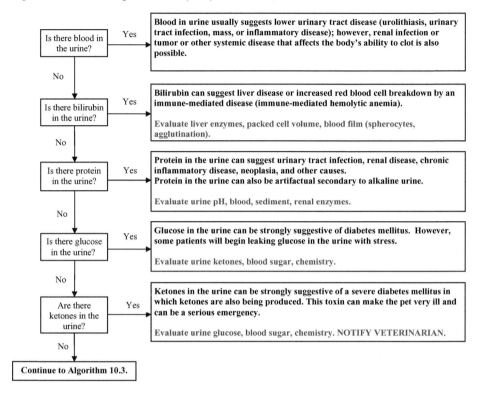

concentrations and glucosuria. Additional testing for other components of the urine that are normally reabsorbed by the proximal convoluted tubule, such as amino acids, is used to confirm these inherited defects in proximal tubular function.

Cats commonly have transient hyperglycemia when excited or stressed. If the hyperglycemia is high enough and persists for long enough there will be spillover of glucose into the urine. This occurrence can make it difficult to differentiate diabetes mellitus from stress in the cat. Serum fructosamine concentration, a test often used to assist in diagnosing diabetes mellitus, will be increased in diabetic cats and be within the reference range in cats with stress hyperglycemia.

Ketonuria

Ketones are produced by animals that are metabolizing fat as their primary source of energy. This usually happens in diabetic animals because glucose is not available for tissue utilization due to lack of insulin. The ketone reagent pad detects two of the three ketones produced with increased fat metabolism: acetoacetate and acetone. The reagent pad reacts most strongly to acetoacetate. The reagent pad does not detect betahydroxybutyrate, the third ketone produced with fat metabolism. Unfortunately, betahydroxybutyrate is the primary ketone produced in diabetic ketoacidosis. Therefore, the ketone reagent pad can show a false negative reaction in some cases. Rarely, ketones are produced in sufficient concentration to cause ketonuria when animals are starved. After insulin therapy, urine ketones can increase significantly because of a shift in the production of ketones from betahydroxybutyrate to acetoacetate.

Bilirubinuria

There are two major types of bilirubin found in the serum: conjugated bilirubin and unconjugated bilirubin. The only type of bilirubin found in the urine is conjugated because the kidney does not filter unconjugated bilirubin. Just as with glucose, there is a renal threshold for bilirubin. As with the glucose threshold, the dog has a lower threshold for bilirubin than the cat. In addition, canine renal tubular epithelial cells can conjugate unconjugated bilirubin and excrete it into the urine. Because of the difference in the renal threshold for bilirubin between the dog and cat, the significance of bilirubin in their urine differs. Dog urine can have trace to 1 + bilirubin with no underlying disease. Although bilirubinuria can be found in normal dog urine, it should not be completely discounted. Bilirubinuria will be seen before hyperbilirubinemia in dogs with early hepatic disease.

In cats, the renal threshold is high enough that hyperbilirubinemia develops before bilirubinuria. Therefore, the presence of bilirubin in feline urine is always significant. The diseases that cause bilirubinuria are the same as those that result in hyperbilirubinemia: liver disease, hemolysis, bile duct obstruction, and sepsis.

Hematuria, Hemoglobinuria, Myoglobinuria

The reagent pad for blood will detect whole blood, lysed blood cells, hemoglobinuria, and myoglobinuria. Differentiating which is present in the urine relies on gross and microscopic examination as well as understanding how the body deals with hemoglobin and myoglobin. Urine samples with a small amount of whole blood (often not detectable grossly) will show a speckled pattern on the blood reagent pad. Hematuria will cause the urine to be red and cloudy. Pigmenturia is the presence of pigments such as hemoglobin and myoglobin. The pigments are soluble; therefore, the urine will be transparent rather than cloudy. Figure 10.2 illustrates the gross appearance of hemoglobinuria and hematuria.

It is difficult to differentiate myoglobinuria from hemoglobinuria by gross

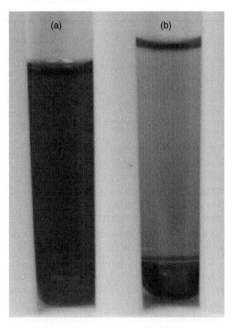

Figure 10.2. Two samples of urine that tested positive for blood on the reagent pad and have been centrifuged. (a) Hemoglobinuria is present. The supernatant remained red after centrifugation and there isn't a red blood cell pellet at the bottom of the tube. (b) Hematuria is present. The supernatant is clear and yellow, and the red cells have been separated into a red pellet at the bottom of the tube.

evaluation of the urine. To differentiate these two, evaluation of the serum is necessary. Hemoglobin is bound to albumin when it is in the plasma; myoglobin is free in the plasma. As a result, myoglobin is rabidly cleared from the blood, and hemoglobin is slowly cleared because the albumin helps keep hemoglobin from being filtered by the kidneys. Patients with hemoglobinuria will have hemoglobinemia. Patients with myoglobinuria will have normal serum or plasma color.

Protein

The reagent pad for protein is most sensitive to albumin. Urine from a patient with normal kidneys usually has no protein present. Very little protein can filter through the glomerulus into the urine. The proximal renal tubular epithelial cells reabsorbed the small amount of protein that does leak into the urine. However, a small amount of protein can be present without any other evidence of renal disease. This can happen with stress, excitement, or strenuous exercise. Pathological proteinuria can be due to glomerular or tubular disease. Injury to the proximal tubule epithelium will prevent the reabsorption of the small amount of protein that normally filters into the urine. The degree of proteinuria seen with tubular disease is usually mild. In contrast, injury to the glomerulus can result in mild to marked proteinuria. The degree of proteinuria is proportional to the severity of the glomerular damage.

Protein can be present in the urine as a result of inflammation in the kidney or bladder, glomerular disease, or renal tubular damage. If the sample is a free-catch collection, the protein can also be from the urethra and prepuce or vagina. Interpretation of the protein reaction depends on the specific gravity and the sediment examination

(Algorithm 10.3). Pyuria, the presence of increased numbers of white blood cells, indicates inflammation, which is usually accompanied by protein as part of the inflammatory process. Quantification of the amount of protein is not helpful when inflammation is present. The proteinuria present with inflammation should resolve once the cause of the inflammation has been treated. However, if there is no evidence of inflammation, proteinuria is a very significant finding in the urinalysis.

When urine is concentrated as it flows through the medulla of the kidney, all of the substances in the urine will increase in concentration as well. Because of this, the protein reaction will be stronger in concentrated urine. A 1 + reaction in a urine sample with a specific gravity of 1.010 is more significant than a 2 + reaction in a urine sample with a specific gravity of 1.035. In many cases, the veterinarian will want to better quantify the degree of proteinuria with further testing. The decision to further quantify the loss of protein in the urine may be prompted by the presence of hypoalbuminemia.

The protein-creatinine ratio provides a quantification of the protein by comparing it to the concentration of creatinine in the urine. The creatinine acts as an internal standard that correlates to the degree of urine concentration. Normal animals will have a very low protein creatinine ratio, <0.5. Significant proteinuria is present when the ratio is > 1.0. Table 10.2 lists the most common diseases that can cause significant proteinuria.

Repeatable detection of small amounts of albumin, **microalbuminuria**, can assist in identifying early renal disease. It is best to test for microalbuminuria as a screen for early renal disease in patients that are at risk. Table 10.3 lists risk factors for development of chronic renal disease. Patients with these risk factors may benefit from screening for persistent early protein loss with a microalbuminuria test.

Algorithm 10.3. Evaluating urine sediment.

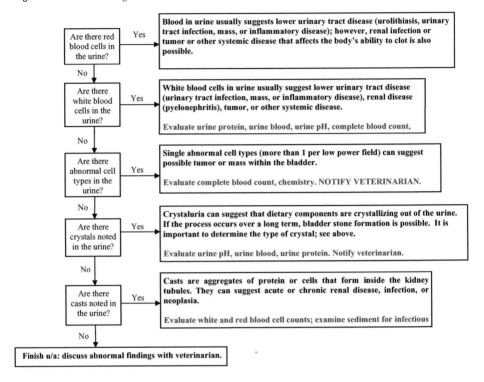

Sediment Examination

Evaluation of the urine sediment is an essential part of the urinalysis. Full interpretation of the chemical reactions for protein and blood require sediment evaluation. Identification of cells, casts, and crystals can assist the veterinarian in developing a differential diagnosis for underlying disease and

Table 10.2. Causes of proteinuria.

Disease	Mechanism	Degree of Proteinuria
Glomerular disease		
Glomerulonephritis	Immune-complex deposition in glomerular capillaries	Mild to moderate
Amyloidosis	Abnormal protein deposition in the glomerulus	Marked
Glomerulopathy	Hereditary defects in the glomerular capillaries	Mild to moderate
Tubular disease		
Fanconi syndrome	Defect in the proximal tubular transports	Mild
Interstitial nephritis	Inhibiting proximal tubular function	Mild to moderate
Drug toxicity	Proximal tubular necrosis	Mild

Table 10.3. Risk factors for development of renal disease.

Chronic inflammatory disease	Dermatitis
	Dental disease
	Immune-mediated disease
Infectious disease	Feline leukemia virus
	Ehrlichiosis
	Heartworm disease
Metabolic disease	Hypertension
	Diabetes mellitus
	Hyperthyroidism
Chronic urinary tract disease	
Neoplasia	

a treatment plan. Urine sediment examination should be both qualitative (identifying specific cast, crystal, and cell types) and quantitative (determining the number of each element per high or low power field).

Urinary Casts

Casts are formed elements that arise in the renal tubules. The appearance of the cast depends on where it forms, how long the cast was present in the tubule, and the contents of the cast. Coarse and granular casts are formed when renal tubular epithelial cells slough into the lumen of the tubule. Initially, the casts will be coarsely granular as the epithelial cells lose their integrity and break up. If the flow of urine is slow, the coarse granular casts will become finely granular as the cell debris continues to degrade while the cast slowly progresses through the tubular system. Waxy casts develop over a long period of time as the lipid component of the cellular debris breaks down forming a large hyaline cast with no recognizable cellular debris. Figure 10.3 illustrates how casts form.

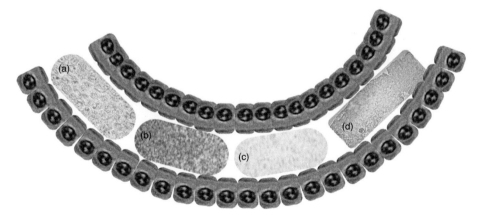

Figure 10.3. Casts are formed by sloughing of cells into the tubule. Initially, the casts are cellular (**a**) As they travel through the tubules they continue to break down into coarsely granular casts (**b**) and then finely granular casts (**c**) and, if they remain in the tubules for long enough, waxy casts (**d**).

Table 10.4. Urinary cast types.

Cast Type	Cause
Hyaline cast	Proteinuria
Granular casts	Renal tubular necrosis
Waxy cast	Chronic renal disease
White cell cast	Inflammation into the renal tubule
Red cell cast	Hemorrhage into the renal tubule

Red blood cell and white blood cell casts form if there is significant inflammation or hemorrhage in the renal tubules. When they are present in the urine, they identify the renal tubule as the site for the inflammation or hemorrhage. They will not be present with cystitis unless there is ascending disease with extension of the inflammatory process from the bladder up through the urethra to the kidney.

Hyaline casts are an indication of increased protein in the urine. Because of their appearance, they are difficult to see on sediment examination unless the condenser is lowered to accentuate contrast in the wet preparation. Table 10.4 lists the individual casts and their causes. In dehydrated animals and animals with renal disease, fluid therapy can result in a transient shower of casts into the urine as urine flow is reestablished. This increase in casts does not mean that there is additional damage to the renal tubules or increased protein loss; it is the result of the increased urine flow "washing" the casts that were present before fluid therapy was initiated out of the tubules.

Urinary Crystals

Urine crystals form when minerals or other constituents precipitate or crystallize in the urine. Crystals can form in the tubules or in the urine. The formation of crystals depends on the concentration of the substance or substances in the urine and the urine pH. Traditionally, crystals can be categorized by the pH of the urine that promotes formation of the crystal. However, although there is an optimum pH for different crystal formation, each crystal type can be seen in acid or alkaline urine, especially if the pH of the urine is near neutral.

Dietary and metabolic factors are the primary elements that promote crystal formation. In addition, bacteria can act as a nidus or center onto which a crystal will grow. Table 10.5 lists the most common crystals, the urine pH they in which they are usually found, and the diseases with which they are associated. The presence of crystals in the urine does not predict the formation of uroliths (urine stones).

Table 10.5. Common urine crystals and associated diseases.

Urine pH	Disease
Neutral to high	Urinary tract infection
Neutral to high	Liver disease, portacaval shunts, normal in dalmatians
Low to neutral	Hyperparathyroidism, hereditary predisposition in miniature schnauzers
Low to neutral	Ethylene glycol intoxication
Not pH-associated	Liver disease, immune-mediated hemolytic anemia
Low to neutral	Hereditary cystinuria

Table 10.6. Cellular elements and associated diseases.

Cell type	Disease
Squamous cells	No clinical significance
Transitional cells	Increased numbers in cystitis, atypical cells associated with neoplasia
Erythrocytes	Cystitis, neoplasia, coagulopathies
Leukocytes	Cystitis, neoplasia, pyelonephritis

Cells

The cells present in urine are leukocytes, erythrocytes, squamous epithelial cells, transitional cells and, rarely, renal tubular epithelial cells. All of these cells can be found in small numbers in urine from clinically normal animals. The method of urine collection has a direct effect on the significance of the cellular elements found in urine. Squamous and transitional epithelial cells usually have little significance, regardless of collection method.

Free-catch urine samples often have low numbers of leukocytes and erythrocytes. If these cells are present in large numbers in a free-catch sample, it is difficult to determine the source of the inflammation or hemorrhage. A catheterized or cystocentesis sample should be obtained. A large number of these cells in a cystocentesis or catheter sample indicate inflammation or hemorrhage within the bladder or kidneys. Cystocentesis can result in small amounts of blood in the urine sample.

Transitional cells increase in number when inflammation of the bladder is present. When inflammation is present, transitional cells can become very atypical and difficult to differentiate from neoplastic cells. If the number or appearance of transitional cells in urine is a concern, the sample should be reviewed by a clinical pathologist. Table 10.6 illustrates the cellular elements found in urine and their association with disease processes.

Adrenal Function and Testing

The adrenal glands are complex organs with multiple functions. They play a central role in the body's response to chronic and acute stress by regulating blood pressure, heart rate, bronchodilatation, electrolyte balance, and blood glucose levels. The adrenal glands are small peanut-shaped glands that sit cranial to both kidneys (Figure 11.1). The glands are composed of two distinctive and separate tissues—the adrenal cortex and the adrenal medulla—and each part has a different function.

Adrenal Cortex

The adrenal cortex is the outer tissue layer responsible for producing different types of steroids for maintenance of blood glucose, electrolytes, and sex hormone production. The cortex has three distinct levels and compromises 75% of the entire gland:

- **Zona granulosa**, which is the outermost area of the cortex and is responsible for

producing a steroid hormone called **aldosterone**, also called a **mineralocorticoid**
- **Zona fasciculata and zona reticularis**, which are the inner regions of the adrenal cortex that produce a prednisone-like steroid called **cortisol** and small amounts of androgens (sex hormones)

Adrenal Medulla

The adrenal medulla is the tissue in the middle of the gland that is responsible for producing **epinephrine** and **norepinephrine** to assist the central nervous system in times of crisis (**"fight or flight response"**). Epinephrine has the following effects on the body:

- Increased heart rate
- Blood vessel constriction → increased blood pressure
- Bronchial airways dilation

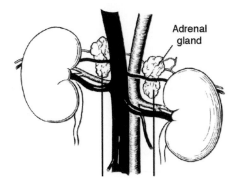

Figure 11.1. The normal position of the adrenal gland in the body.

- Decreased intestinal secretion and movement
- Pupil dilation

Adrenal Function

In general, the adrenal gland has three primary functions that regulate the body's response to stress:

- Cortisol production
- Mineralocorticoid production
- Epinephrine production

Adrenal-Pituitary Axis: Cortisol Production

Cortisol is produced by the adrenal cortex to take protein and fat and turn them into glucose in times of low blood glucose. The three-step process is controlled by a small gland in the brain called the **pituitary gland**, also called the "master gland":

1. When the brain senses low blood glucose, the pituitary gland releases **adrenocorticotrophic hormone (ACTH)** to stimulate the adrenal gland to produce cortisol.

2. ACTH is released into the bloodstream where it encounters specific protein receptors in the adrenal cortex that stimulate the release of cortisol into the blood. The circulating cortisol stimulates the conversion of protein and fat into glucose, primarily in the liver.

3. As cortisol levels increase in the blood, the pituitary decreases the amount of ACTH released. **This is called a negative feedback loop** (Figure 11.2).

Adrenal Cortex: Mineralocorticoid Production

The adrenal cortex also produces a mineralocorticoid called **aldosterone** that is responsible for the reabsorption of sodium and excretion of potassium in the distal convoluted tubules in the kidney (Figure 11.3). Without this hormone, the renal medulla is unable to maintain the high sodium gradient and thus cannot concentrate urine. **This hormone above all other adrenal hormones is needed for normal handling of stress and electrolyte maintenance. Without sufficient levels of this hormone, an animal can develop a life-threatening Addisonian crisis:**

- Aldosterone is necessary for the **maintenance of the sodium/potassium balance** within the body. Sodium is the electrolyte found in highest concentrations in the serum and the extracellular fluid in the body. Potassium is found in the highest concentrations inside the cell.
- All muscle contraction and nerve depolarization require sodium and potassium to switch places to produce the electrical impulse necessary for the action (Figure 11.4).
- When the normal sodium and potassium concentrations in the cells and blood are altered, the body has a harder time producing normal electrical activity, and the patient becomes weakened, with muscle fasiculations and

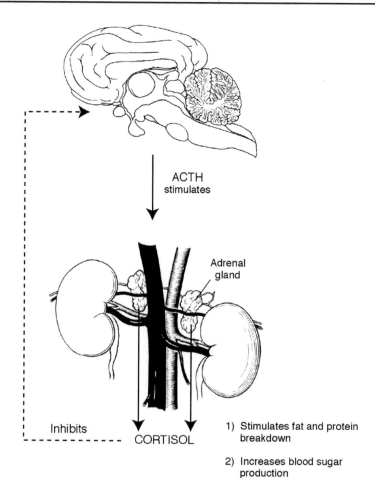

Figure 11.2. ACTH stimulates the release of cortisol. Cortisol then stimulates production of blood glucose from fats and muscle, while also decreasing the production of ACTH. This type of model is called a **negative feedback loop.**

abnormally slow heart rhythms. Severely affected animals can develop a life threatening condition, called an **Addisonian crisis.**

Adrenal Cortex: Epinephrine Production

As mentioned earlier, epinephrine is the hormone associated with the fight or flight response. It is closely linked to the sympathetic nervous system, a division of the autonomic nervous system of the body. Epinephrine is secreted when an animal is threatened and produces the following changes in the body:

- Increased heart rate
- Increased Blood pressure
- Bronchodilatation to increase airflow into the body

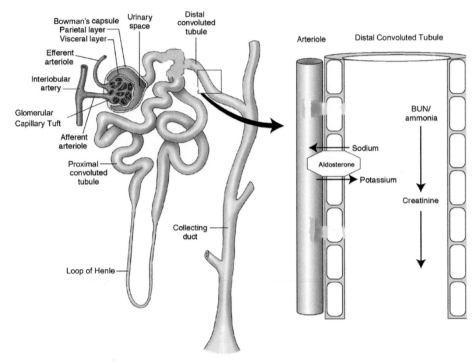

Figure 11.3. Sodium is reabsorbed and potassium excreted in the distal convoluted tubules due to the action of aldosterone.

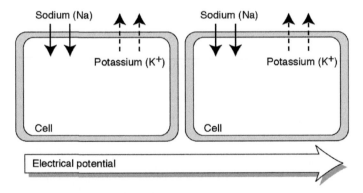

Figure 11.4. Sodium/potassium exchange occurs within the cell to produce an electrical wave. These electrical waves are key to normal neurological, cardiovascular, and muscular actions. Without proper concentrations of sodium and potassium, the patient will experience severe weakness.

- Stopping intestinal movement and salivation
- Pupil dilation

Evaluating the Patient with Adrenal Disease

Three types of adrenal disease are commonly seen in general practice; hyperadrenocorticism (Cushing's disease), hypoadrenocorticism (Addison's disease), and pheochromocytoma.

Hyperadrenocorticism (Cushing's Disease)

Hyperadrenocorticism is an overproduction of cortisol caused by primary adrenal or pituitary disease.

Clinical Signs of Adrenal Disease

The following are clinical signs of adrenal disease:

- **Chronic infection/skin disease:** Thinning of the skin, generalized increased pigmentation, hair loss (alopecia), rash, or plaques on the skin
- **Polydipsia, polyuria, and polyphagia:** Increased thirst, urination, and appetite.
- **Chronic skin disease:** Due to long-term exposure to chronic steroidal medication, patients can have symmetrical hair loss on both sides of the abdomen, thinning of the skin or fragile skin, and increased deposition of pigment.
- **Abdominal distention:** Due to increased protein catabolism from long-term steroidal effects, the abdominal musculature begins to thin and the patient appears pot-bellied (Figure 11.5).
- **Panting:** Panting is often reported as a side effect to increased steroidal medication or production.
- **Lethargy:** Generally, clinical hyperadrenocortical patients have decreased energy and are more depressed.

Forms of Hyperadrenocorticism

There are three forms of hyperadrenocorticism:

- Pituitary-dependent hyperadrenocorticism (PDH)

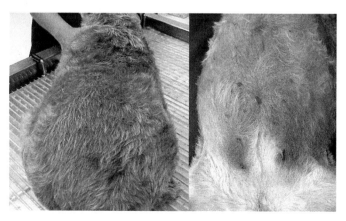

Figure 11.5. Image of a patient with distended or pot-bellied abdomen due to long-term affects of steroids decreasing abdominal musculature.

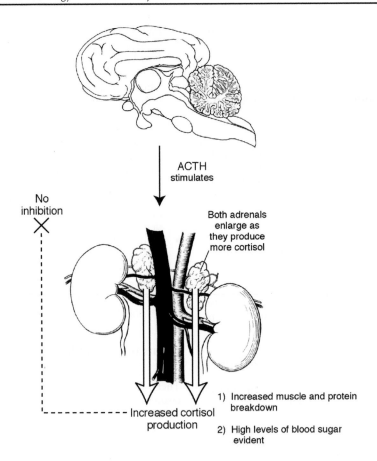

ACTH
stimulates

No
inhibition
X

Both adrenals
enlarge as
they produce
more cortisol

1) Increased muscle and protein breakdown

Increased cortisol production

2) High levels of blood sugar evident

Figure 11.6.   Pituitary-dependent form of hyperadrenocorticism (Cushing's disease). In this case, microscopic tumors of the pituitary overproduce ACTH, producing bilaterally enlarged adrenal glands, which then overproduce cortisol, producing Cushing's disease.

- Adrenal neoplasia
- Iatrogenic hyperadrenocorticism

Pituitary-Dependent Hyperadrenocorticism (PDH)

This form of the disease is caused by a pituitary tumor, which produces excessive amounts of ACTH and causes overstimulation of both adrenal glands; this results in constant production of cortisol. These tu-mors do not respond to the negative feed-back of increased circulating cortisol. If the pituitary tumor becomes large enough, neu-rologic disease can be seen (i.e., seizures) (Figure 11.6).

Adrenal Neoplasia

A less common cause of hyperadrenocorti-cism is a tumor of the adrenal cortex that produces excessive amounts of cortisol. In

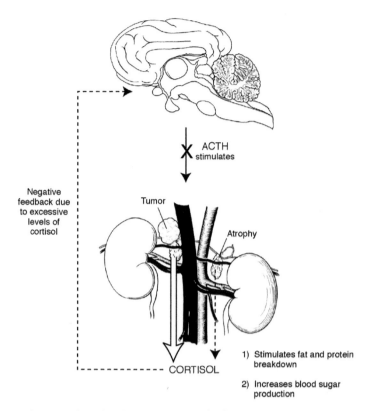

Figure 11.7. With a tumor of the adrenal cortex, the affected gland overproduces cortisol irrespective of the ACTH in the blood. The increasing blood cortical concentration decreases ACTH production, causing secondary atrophy of the unaffected adrenal gland.

this case, one adrenal gland is usually enlarged and the other is small (atrophied). The high concentration of cortisol and secondary increase of glucose in the blood cause a decrease in secretion of ACTH by the pituitary through the negative feedback loop. Because there is decreased circulating ACTH, the other adrenal gland is small and atrophied (Figure 11.7).

Iatrogenic Hyperadrenocorticism

Long-term administration of exogenous steroids (i.e., prednisone) can disrupt the normal negative feedback loop by causing suppression of ACTH section by the pituitary gland. The decreased circulating ACTH causes atrophy of both adrenal glands. The exogenous steroids produce clinical signs similar to the other forms of hyperadrenocorticism. However, if the exogenous steroids are discontinued abruptly, the patient develops signs of decreased adrenal function and may produce a life-threatening Addisonian crisis. This consequence of iatrogenic hyperadrenocortism can be avoided with a slow withdrawal of the exogenous steroids.

It is very difficult to diagnose most forms of hyperadrenocorticism with routine blood work. Changes in the CBC and chemistry profile can support a diagnosis of hyperadrenocorticism but should not be considered diagnostic for the disease. Advanced diagnostic tests are needed to confirm the diagnosis of hyperadrenocorticism and differentiate primary pituitary disease from adrenal disease (see Figure 11.10, later in this chapter). The choice of a diagnostic protocol to evaluate for hyperadrenocorticism depends on the preference of the clinician and the history and clinical findings of the patient.

Routine Diagnostics for Hyperadrenocorticism

Serum Color

As discussed previously, it is important for the technical team to always evaluate and record serum color as part of routine diagnostic testing.

Patients with many forms of endocrine disease, including hyperadrenocorticism, can have lipemic serum (see Figure 11.8).

It is important to note that Lipemia can also be seen as an artifact when a blood sample is collected from a pet that has just recently eaten. In general, a fast of 12 hours is recommended to eliminate postprandial lipemia. If lipemia persists greater than 12 hours, the patient should be evaluated for diseases that may produce altered fat metabolism.

Complete Blood Count

The complete blood count can be normal; however, a **stress leukogram** is commonly seen. A stress leukogram is characterized by the following:

- A slight increase in white blood cells count

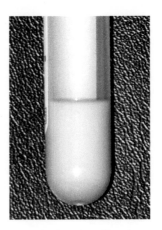

Figure 11.8. Is this lipemia artifactual or suggestive of a disease state? Endocrine diseases that affect fat metabolism (i.e., hyperadrenocorticism, diabetes mellitus, and hypothyroidism) may result in lipemic serum. It is important for the technical team to record changes in the gross appearance of serum samples. In addition, suggesting underlying disease, this change will affect in-house clinical chemistry values.

- An increased neutrophil count
- A decreased lymphocyte count
- An increased monocyte count in the dog

Chemistry

Changes in a routine chemistry profile can be extremely variable. **There is no absolute test for adrenal disease on a routine chemistry profile; however, the following sections review some commonly observed changes.**

Alkaline Phosphatase

Alkaline phosphatase refers to a large number of intracellular enzymes that are present within the liver, intestine, bone, kidneys, and placenta (see Chapter 6). Serum alkaline phosphatase concentration is one of the most common changes seen in the chemistry profile of patients with hyperadrenocorticism. Increased circulating steroids increase the production and release of alkaline phosphatase by hepatocytes. This process is called **induction**.

It is important to note that patients with hyperadrenocorticism can have normal levels of alkaline phosphatase and still have significant disease.

ALT and AST

Chronic stimulation of hepatocytes by circulating corticosteroids causes excessive accumulation of glycogen and can result in hepatocellular damage with release of ALT and AST.

Cholesterol

Increased cholesterol can be seen with hyperadrenocorticism due to increased fat mobilization.

Blood Glucose

Animals with chronically high levels of cortisol can be **hyperglycemic.** Blood glucose in nondiabetic animals can range from 200–300 mg/dL. In 20% of hyperadrenocorticism patients, diabetes can occur due to corticosteroid-induced insulin resistance.

Urinalysis

The ability of the kidneys to concentrate urine can be affected by increased circulating corticosteroids. Animals are usually **hyposthenuric with urine specific gravities under 1.008.** Corticosteroids inhibit the actions of the pituitary hormone ADH (antidiuretic hormone), the hormone that regulates reabsorption of water in the kidneys. In addition, if the disease is chronic enough, loss of sodium in the medullary region of the kidneys will decrease the osmotic gradient necessary for reabsorption of water (see Chapter 5).

Advanced Diagnostics for Hyperadrenocorticism

The diagnosis of adrenal dysfunction requires special diagnostic tests that evaluate the responsiveness of the adrenal-pituitary axis. There are several diagnostic tests available; each has its own value in evaluating a patient for abnormal adrenal function (see Figure 11.10, later in this chapter). The following sections review diagnostic tests commonly used to support a diagnosis of hyperadrenocorticism.

Urine Cortisol/Creatinine Ratio Test

In animals with hyperadrenocorticism or chronic stress, excess cortisol is excreted by the kidneys increasing the concentration of cortisol in comparison to creatinine in the urine. A single urine sample is obtained and submitted to a reference laboratory. Results can include the following:

- Increased levels of cortisol raise the cortisol/creatinine ratio >1.
- A normal urine cortisol/creatinine ratio rules out Cushing's disease.
- An elevated cortisol/creatinine ratio supports, but is not diagnostic for, hyperadrenocorticism. Any disease associated with chronic stress will increase the cortisol/creatinine ratio.

Therefore, this test is a good screening test to rule out hyperadrenocorticism.

ACTH Stimulation Test

The following procedure is used for this test:

1. The patient is fasted for 12 hours and a blood sample is taken for a **prestimulation cortisol level.**

2. ACTH is given, either intramuscularly or intravenously, depending on the form of ACTH administered.
3. 1 or 2 hours later (depending on the form of ACTH administered), a blood sample is taken for a **poststimulation cortisol level.**

Patients with hyperadrenocorticism show an exaggerated increase (far above the normal response to ACTH) in blood cortisol concentration after stimulation of the adrenal gland; this response is due to their enlarged hypertrophic adrenal glands. Although this test is helpful in diagnosing hyperadrenocorticism, it does not distinguish between pituitary-dependent disease and an adrenal tumor.

Low-Dose Dexamethasone Suppression Test

The following procedure is used for this test:

1. The patient is fasted for 12 hours and a blood sample is taken for a **pretest cortisol level.**
2. A low dose of dexamethasone is injected intravenously.
3. 6 **and** 8 hours after injection, blood samples are taken for additional cortisol concentration determinations.

In the normal animal, cortisol concentration should be suppressed through the negative feedback system, decreasing ACTH secretion and lowering cortisol production by the adrenal glands. A normal animal will suppress its blood cortisol concentration by 50% 6 to 8 hours after the initial dexamethasone injection.

In the patient with hyperadrenocorticism, there is no suppression of the cortisol after 8 hours.

With pituitary disease, the pituitary tumors will not decrease ACTH secretion when faced with increasing cortisol or cortisol-like drug concentrations in the blood. The abnormal pituitary tissue does not respond to negative feedback.

Adrenal tumors do not depend on ACTH from the pituitary for production of cortisol. Therefore, they do not decrease cortisol production when faced with decreasing blood ACTH concentration.

This test is an excellent screening for Cushing's disease; however, this test does not distinguish between pituitary dependent disease and an adrenal tumor.

High-Dose Dexamethasone Suppression Test

This test is done to differentiate between adrenal or pituitary forms of the disease after the low-dose dexamethasone suppression test or the ACTH stimulation test have confirmed the diagnosis of hyperadrenocorticism.

The following procedure is used for this test:

1. The patient is fasted for 12 hours and a blood sample is taken for a **pretest cortisol level.**
2. A high dosage of dexamethasone is injected intravenously.
3. 6 and 8 hours after injection, blood samples are taken for additional cortisol concentration determinations.

In the patient with pituitary-dependent disease, the pituitary tumor will decrease ACTH production in the face of a higher dexamethasone dose. The decreased ACTH secretion in turn causes decreased cortisol release from the adrenal glands and blood cortical goes down (is suppressed).

In the patient with an **adrenal tumor,** blood cortical concentration will not suppress in response to a higher dexamethasone

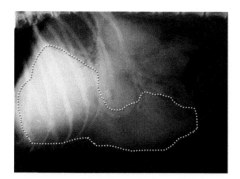

Figure 11.9. An x-ray image of an enlarged liver secondary to possible chronic steroid exposure. Neoplasia, infectious disease, or other forms of liver disease can also cause liver enlargement.

dose because it is not a responsive change in blood ACTH concentration.

Additional Diagnostic Tests for Hyperadrenocorticism

Radiology

Abdominal radiographs are used to assess organ enlargement (i.e., **hepatomegaly**) or potential adrenal masses in patients with clinical signs of hyperadrenocorticism. Although many diseases can produce organ enlargement, chronic increased blood corticosteroid concentrations can produce an increased liver mass (Figure 11.9).

Blood Pressure

One of the most common causes of canine hypertension is hyperadrenocorticism. It is recommended that patients being evaluated for hyperadrenocorticism have systolic blood pressure evaluated. Dogs with blood pressure persistently >150–160 mm Hg should be followed and may require treatment.

Ultrasound

When hyperadrenocorticism is considered as the likely diagnosis by review of routine clinical diagnostic tests, advanced diagnostic screening tests (i.e., ACTH response test, low-dose dexamethasone suppression test), abdominal ultrasound imaging can help confirm bilaterally enlarged adrenal glands or an adrenal mass. Ultrasound can help detect the following:

- **Pituitary-dependent disease:** With this form of the disease, abdominal ultrasound can help indicate moderate (1–2 × normal size) enlargement of **both adrenal glands** due to increased ACTH production from the pituitary gland.
- **Adrenal tumor:** With this form of the disease, abdominal ultrasound can help indicate moderate enlargement of one adrenal gland and atrophy of the other gland secondary to negative feedback of increased Cortisol concentrations and decreased ACTH levels.

Text Box 11.1
Discussing Clinical Diagnostic Tests for Hyperadrenocorticism with the Client

- The veterinarian is recommending initial baseline blood and urinalysis diagnostics to help evaluate your pet for Cushing's disease, also known as hyperadrenocorticism. This disease is caused by an overproduction of steroids by the adrenal Gland.
- Although routine blood work and urinalysis will not absolutely confirm Cushing, these diagnostic tests will help indicate whether further testing is needed to confirm or rule out the disease. Further, the routine diagnostic tests will allow the veterinarian to assess for other organ dysfunction that could occur secondary to Cushing's disease (i.e., diabetes mellitus, liver disease).

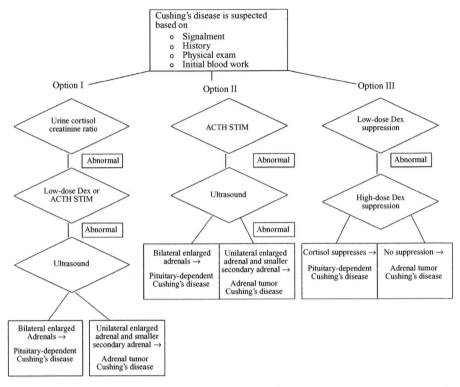

Figure 11.10. The decision tree gives team members an overview of the clinical diagnostic protocols that may be used to help confirm or rule out hyperadrenocorticism. *This diagram is not meant to help diagnose the disease, but to understand the complexity of testing to help discuss diagnostic options with the client.*

- If Cushing's disease is suspected, advanced diagnostic tests and abdominal imaging may be needed.
- The type of the disease (pituitary vs. adrenal) must be diagnosed in order for an appropriate treatment protocol to be recommended.

Long-Term Monitoring of the Patient with Hyperadrenocorticism

Treatment protocols largely focus on destroying the adrenal cell layer that produces cortisol or decreasing the body's ability to produce steroid hormones. Controlling the disease requires a lifelong commitment by owners to monitor their pets for recurrence of physical symptoms and routine reevaluation of blood work.

Over time, patients with hyperadrenocorticism can develop diabetes mellitus, hypertension, secondary liver disease (**steroid hepatopathy**), decreased ability to fight infection (immunosuppression), muscle loss, and skin changes from chronic steroidal exposure. In addition, patients may develop hypoadrenocorticism, because medical treatment of the disease destroys the adrenal cells that produce both cortisol and aldosterone (see the section "Hypoadrenocorticism," later in this chapter).

Chronic Infection/Skin Pathology	Diabetes Mellitus (20% of all Cushing's Patients)

Client–Thinning of the skin, increased pigmentation, generalized hair loss (alopecia), rash or plaques in the skin
With Concern Diagnostics Can Include

- ACTH or adrenal function testing
- Thyroid level
- Complete blood count and chemistry

Client–Increased thirst & urination
With Concern Diagnostics Can Include

- Serial U/a
- Serial blood sugar
- Fructosamine

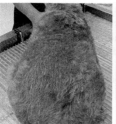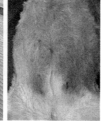

Hypoadrenocortical Patients (From Treatment)

Client–

- Weakness
- Vomiting, diarrhea
- Collapsing
- Bradycardia

With Concern Diagnostics Can Include

- Electrolytes
- ACTH Response test
- Fructosamine

Liver Disease (Steroid Hepatopathy)	Hypertension

Client–Vomiting, diarrhea, weight loss, jaundice, weakeness
With Concern Diagnostics Can Include

- Chemistry–lever profile
- Bile acids
- Ultrasound

Client–Weakness, "...patient acting old or not right,..." blindness, exercise intolerance
With Concern Diagnostics Can Include

- Blood pressure

Figure 11.11. Illustration of secondary disease, physical symptoms, and clinical diagnostic tests that are evaluated when treating and monitoring the Patient with hyperadrenocorticism.

Hospital teams should consider and discuss these concerns with clients and make sure that the owners are aware of physical signs that could suggest changes in the patient's disease status and of routine clinical monitoring of patients (Figure 11.11). Suggested clinical pathology testing for the long-term management of the patient with hyperadrenocorticism includes the tests reviewed in the following sections.

Complete Blood Count and Chemistry Profile

The medical team should evaluate for changes in the CBC that suggest inflammatory or infectious disease. Further, the chemistry should be evaluated for changes in liver enzymes that may suggest liver in-

jury, changes in electrolytes to monitor for any changes that could suggest hypoadrenocorticism, and changes in blood glucose concentration that could suggest early signs of diabetes mellitus.

ACTH Stimulation Test

This clinical diagnostic test is used at regular intervals to evaluate the patient's response to medication and to make sure the patient is responding to medication by suppressing the production of cortisol but has not developed clinical hypoadrenocorticism (Addison's disease). Based the results of the test, the veterinarian can change medication or level of medication to maximize control of the disease.

Blood Pressure Evaluation

If the patient continues to remain poorly controlled by medication, routine evaluation of blood pressure should be monitored. If a patient becomes hypertensive, medications to control the hypertension (see Chapter 5) may be added.

Bile Acids/Abdominal Ultrasound

If the patient begins to show physical symptoms of liver disease or if there are changes in the blood work to suggest liver damage, bile acid assays are often recommended to assess liver function (see chapter 6). If liver function is affected, often abdominal ultrasound and ultrasound-guided biopsy may be elected to help identify the type of liver injury.

Hypoadrenocorticism

The second form of adrenal disease is **hypoadrenocorticism (Addison's disease)**, a decreased production of aldosterone and/or cortisol by the adrenal gland. The lack of aldosterone inhibits the kidney's ability to retain sodium and excrete potassium. The lack of cortisol inhibits normal release of blood glucose in times of crisis or response to stress. Addison's disease is caused by destruction of the adrenal cortex.

Disease Processes

The following sections review several disease processes that can result in destruction or loss of the cortical tissue.

Idiopathic

In most cases of hypoadrenocorticism, the exact cause of the loss of cortical tissue is unknown. The most likely disease process is thought to be immune-mediated destruction of the cortical tissue.

Iatrogenic

As discussed in the previous section on hyperadrenocorticism, chronic administration of steroids can result in loss of adrenal cortical tissue due to atrophy. When the exogenous steroids are abruptly discontinued, the patient may show clinical signs of hypoadrenocorticism. In addition, the drugs used to treat hyperadrenocorticism can cause necrosis of the cortical tissue. If the necrosis is extensive, hypoadrenocorticism will develop and the patient will then need to be treated for Addison's disease.

Granulomatous Disease

Several infectious diseases, primarily fungal, can affect the adrenal cortical tissue. In these cases, the cortical tissue is replaced by inflammatory cells that form multiple granulomas.

Neoplasia

Cancer can spread from other organs (metastasize) to the adrenal gland or invade from the adrenal medulla and destroy the normal adrenal cortical tissue.

Forms of Hypoadrenocorticism

There are two forms of hypoadrenocorticism. The most common type is called primary Addison's disease. This disease results from a decrease production of aldosterone and cortisol due to lack of adrenal cortical tissue. These patients lose the ability to retain sodium and excrete potassium, produce glucose when the patient is hypoglycemic, and respond to stress. Patients suffering from the primary form of hypoadrenocorticism can develop a life-threatening crisis (Addisonian crisis) from their inability to balance sodium and potassium concentrations in blood and tissues.

The second form of Addison's disease (atypical Addison's disease) occurs when the patient lose the ability to produce cortisol only. These patients have a decreased ability to produce glucose when hypoglycemic and respond to stress, but they do not typically present with life-threatening electrolyte imbalance.

Diagnostic Tests for Hypoadrenocorticism

Routine blood and urine diagnostic tests are often more helpful in evaluating the patient's hypoadrenocorticism compared to hyperadrenocorticism. The following changes in routine blood work are often seen in the patient with hypoadrenocorticism.

Chemistry

Electrolyte Imbalance

With hypoadrenocorticism:

- The body is not able to reabsorb sodium and excrete potassium.
- The patient has decreased levels of sodium and increased concentration of potassium.
- The sodium/potassium ratio is decreased.
- The normal sodium/potassium ratio is >25:1 (Na:K); a ratio of <23:1 is suggestive of Addison's disease.

Hypoglycemia

Occasionally, patients in an Addisonian crisis will have a significantly decreased blood glucose concentration. Blood glucose <60 mg/dL should be treated as a life-threatening emergency (see Chapter 15).

Azotemia

When patients are admitted in an Addisonian crisis, they are weak, dehydrated, and often hypotensive. These factors slow glomerular filtration of the blood (see Chapter 5) and increased BUN and creatinine concentrations. Usually, the elevation in BUN and creatinine concentration is mild to moderate.

Urinalysis

The ability of the kidneys to concentrate urine is affected by the decreased sodium in the renal medulla (see Chapter 5). Animals are usually **hyposthenuric with a urine specific gravity of 1.008 to 1.012. It is important to understand the exception to the rule for differentiating prerenal from renal azotemia: Addisonian patients are azotemic with dilute urine but do not have primary renal disease.** Once controlled with proper medication, these patients will be able to concentrate their urine and filter their blood properly.

ACTH Stimulation Test

The ACTH response test is necessary to evaluate the adrenal glands' response to ACTH and confirm the diagnosis of hypoadrenocorticism:

- The normal response produces a measurable moderate rise in blood cortisol 2 hours after administration of ACTH.
- In the patient with hypoadrenocorticism, there is no response to cortisol levels after administration of ACTH.

Text Box 11.2
Discussing Clinical Diagnostic Tests for
Hypoadrenocorticism with the Client

• The veterinarian is recommending initial
  routine blood and urinalysis tests to help
  evaluate your pet for Addison's disease,
  which is the lack of production of steroids
  from the adrenal gland.
• The veterinarian will evaluate changes in
  the urine and the blood electrolytes (i.e.,
  sodium and potassium) that suggest an
  imbalance in the normal reabsorption of
  sodium and excretion of potassium from
  the body.
• If Addison's disease is suspected,
  advanced diagnostic testing may be
  recommended.

Evaluating a patient for atypical Addison's disease is more difficult; these patients produce enough aldosterone to maintain normal electrolyte concentrations. In
addition, patients suffering from this form
of the disease have mild signs of chronic
anorexia, vomiting, weakness, and other
general clinical signs. Often, veterinarians
include ACTH stimulation testing in the diagnostic process for patients suffering from
symptoms of chronic vomiting, diarrhea,
and anorexia. Patients suffering from atypical Addison's disease will show no response
to ACTH.

Pheochromocytoma

The third and final adrenal gland disease is **pheochromocytoma**, cancer of the
adrenal medulla, the epinephrine-producing
tissue of the adrenal gland. This rare type
of cancer can cause severe hypertension,
rapid heart rate, weakness, and eventually
death. Except for having potential severe
life-threatening hypertension, these patients
show little change in their clinical diagnostic database.

12 Blood Gas

Every animal requires chemical reactions to produce energy, fight off infection, or handle electrolyte abnormalities. A simple example of a common metabolic reaction is the conversion of sugar (glucose) into energy. The following is the basic formula for this reaction:

$$C_6H_{12}O_6 \text{ (Sugar)} + H_2O + O_2 \xrightarrow[\text{pH } 7.35-7.45]{} \text{Energy} + CO_2$$

In order for this reaction to occur properly, the body must have adequate levels of blood sugar, oxygen, and a proper blood pH. If one of these factors is limited, the production of energy is affected. An excellent example is when people begin to exercise; they may limit the amount of oxygen needed to produce essential energy. In this situation, the patient begins to anaerobically (without oxygen) convert sugar into energy and lactic acid. Not only is this not as efficient a way to produce energy, lactic acid lowers the body's pH and produces an acidotic state.

$$C_6H_{12}O_6 \text{ (Sugar)} + \text{no } O_2$$
$$\xrightarrow[\text{anaerobic fermentation}]{} \text{Energy (decreased)}$$
$$+ \text{Lactic Acid} + CO_2$$

People affected by lactic acidosis become weak, anorexic, nauseous, and potentially shocky.

When factors produce a change in blood pH, the normal body's reaction can be slowed and the patient can become ill. Acidosis is defined as a decrease in plasma bicarbonate concentration (HCO_3) or an increase in carbon dioxide (CO_2) in a patient. Bicarbonate is a natural buffer that helps to maintain neutral pH when blood pH becomes acidic; loss of blood bicarbonate levels is generally associated with conditions producing metabolic disease (**metabolic acidosis**).

Carbon dioxide is an acid that is produced as the body metabolizes sugar to form energy; increase in blood carbon dioxide

167

levels are generally associated with disease that affects gas exchange in the lungs (**respiratory acidosis**). These changes in chemical population move the normal blood pH away from its neutral pH 7.35–7.45 into an acidic pH. With acidic pH, the body's chemical reactions cannot function normally and the patient becomes weakened, sick, and debilitated.

Etiology

Metabolic acidosis occurs as pH is lowered in the bloodstream. This occurs from a combination of factors, which include a loss of bicarbonate due to a loss of body fluids, an addition of an abnormal acid to the fluid pool, or decreased renal secretion of acid (Figure 12.1). The following are common examples of metabolic acidosis:

- **Loss of HCO₃-rich fluids:** diarrhea (excessive), hypoadrenocorticism

- **Acid added to body:** diabetic ketoacidosis, lactic acidosis, antifreeze intoxication (ethylene glycol), snail bait poisoning (paraldehyde)
- **Decreased acid secretion:** renal disease (renal tubular disease)

Metabolic acidosis can affect any species, breed, sex, or age of animal. The patient with metabolic acidosis may have a history of a chronic disease that can reduce the body's ability to excrete toxin (i.e., diabetes, renal disease, and hypoadrenocorticism), a history of exposure to toxins (antifreeze, snail bait, aspirin overdose), or a disease that produces excessive vomiting/diarrhea (i.e., parvo, pancreatitis, HE, etc.). Metabolic acidosis can be subtle, producing a large variety of signs but, in general, the patient will show the following:

- Nausea
- Weakness
- V/D
- Dehydration

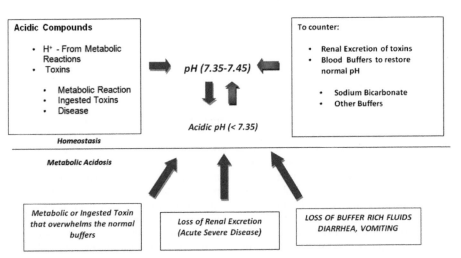

Figure 12.1. An illustration of causative factors that produce acidosis. In the healthy patient, acidic compounds, such as hydrogen ions from metabolic reactions and toxins, lower blood pH. However renal excretion of toxins and normal blood buffers counter this pH drop and maintain normal levels. In the metabolically ill patient, overwhelming toxin load, the loss of renal excretion (i.e. dehydration, renal tubular acidosis), and loss of buffer-rich fluids (i.e., diarrhea and vomiting), overwhelm the patient and produce a severe metabolic acidosis.

- Cardiac arrhythmias
- Shock
- Hyperventilation (body's response to acidosis → decreasing CO_2 levels)

Altered breathing patterns or hyperventilation can occur as decreases in pH stimulate the body to remove other acid sources. The body then increases respiration to remove carbon dioxide, producing a hyperventilation respiratory pattern. This pattern of abnormal breathing and decreased CO_2 in the face of acidosis is called a **compensating metabolic acidosis**. It is important to note that even with a patient's ability to lower CO_2, this may not be sufficient to control the acidosis (see below).

Respiratory acidosis is a buildup of carbon dioxide due to improper oxygen exchange in the body or decreased oxygenation of the patient (Figure 12.2). The following are the most common causes:

- Inadequate oxygenation from anesthesia (i.e., decreased ventilation or poor ventilation)
- Anesthesia of a metabolically ill patient—i.e., gastrodilatation volvulus (GDV)
- A patient with severe pneumonia

The following are common physical symptoms:

- Decreased metabolic reactions
- Cardiac arrhythmia
- Decreased ability to oxygenate tissue
- Shock

If either form of acidosis is not aggressively treated, the patient can become weak, ill, nauseous, or prone to cardiac arrhythmia or shock, and may die.

Blood gas is generally included as part of a clinical diagnostic baseline dependent upon the patient, its medical history, and the physical symptoms. With metabolic acidosis, blood gases are generally evaluated as a part of clinical diagnostic baseline (i.e., complete blood count, chemistry, electrolytes, blood gases, and urinalysis). Further, it can also be utilized as a diagnostic or prognostic indicator to determine whether the patient is responding to treatment, to obtain a differential disease list, and to outline treatment options. With metabolic acidosis, the clinical diagnostic parameters are blood pH, partial pressure of CO_2 (pCO_2), anion gap, and base excess. This can be obtained through a venous sample by normal collection methods.

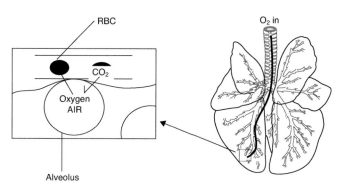

Figure 12.2. Illustration of gas exchange at the alveolar level. In this image, oxygen is breathed in through the trachea, the bronchi, into the alveolus. The enlarged drawing of the alveolus shows that oxygen is exchanged for carbon dioxide in the blood. With respiratory acidosis, this process does not occur and CO_2 levels increase in the blood.

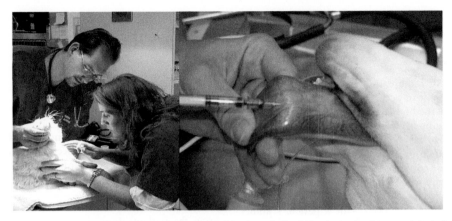

Figure 12.3. With signs of metabolic acidosis, a venous blood sample should be obtained and the sample included as part of a diagnostic baseline. With signs of respiratory acidosis, an arterial sample is indicated. For anesthesia patients, the sublingual artery is often a good choice.

With respiratory acidosis, blood gases are generally evaluated with anesthetic patients under long-term surgical procedures, animals on mechanical ventilators, and animals during emergency surgery with possible underlying metabolic issues (i.e., GDV—endotoxic shock). To evaluate the patient for respiratory acidosis, the clinical diagnostic parameters are blood pH, pCO_2, pO_2, HCO_3, and % saturated oxygen level. In anesthetized patients, an arterial blood stick of a sublingual vessel offers easy exposure to a small arterial (Figure 12.3).

Once blood samples are obtained there is a simple four-step algorithm to evaluate a patient for acidosis (Algorithm 12.1).

This process helps to determine whether the patient is acidotic, the cause of the acidosis, the prognosis, possible differential diseases that can cause the acidosis, and the outline treatment options.

Step 1: Identify Acidosis

An acidotic patient has a pH <7.35. This factor alone designates whether the patient is acidotic and may require treatment. A patient with pH >7.45 is alkalotic. In general, acidotic patients require evaluation, treating, and monitoring. In general, alkalotic patients, except those receiving sodium bicarbonate therapies, will not require treatment or monitoring.

Step 2: Determine the Type of Acidosis

To determine the cause of the acidosis, the medical team must evaluate the partial pressure of carbon dioxide (pCO_2). With an acidotic patient:

- **Decreased pCO_2 (<35 mm HG) or normal pCO_2 (34–40 mm HG)** indicates a primary metabolic acidosis. Because CO_2 levels are low to normal, the patient is becoming acidotic due to increased blood toxins, decreased filtration, or loss of bicarbonate-rich fluids.
- **Low pCO_2 (<35 mm HG)** indicates a primary metabolic acidosis with respiratory compensation. The patient is trying to expel carbon dioxide at an increased rate to help counter the metabolic acidification. This usually presents with a patient with altered or abnormal respiratory cycle (i.e., hyperventilating). **However, this process is not always enough to reverse the acidosis.**

Algorithm 12.1. Causes of acidosis.

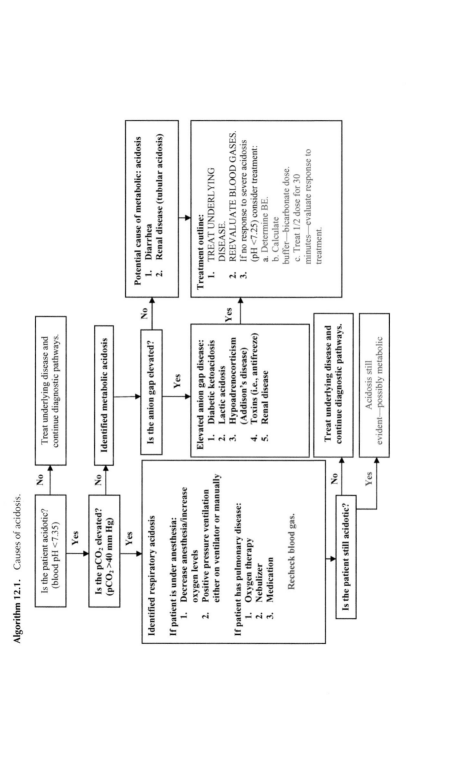

- **Normal pCO_2 (34–40 mm HG)** indicates a primary metabolic acidosis without respiratory compensation.
- **Increased pCO_2 (>40 mm HG)** indicates a primary respiratory acidosis. The patient has decreased ability to exchange gases at the alveolar level and carbon dioxide is building up in the bloodstream. Carbon dioxide is an acid and leads to a lowering of the blood pH.

Step 3: Develop a Differential List for Metabolic Acidosis

If dealing with a metabolic acidotic patient, the next step is to develop a potential differential list for the cause of the acidosis. In many situations, general blood work can be ambiguous and, by evaluating all components of blood gas, the medical team may be able to isolate a cause of the disease process.

To do this, the medical team must evaluate **the anion gap (AG)**. Patients have positively and negatively charged ions that help to regulate electrical impulses, moderate chemical reactions, and aid in multiple metabolic functions. The typical measured ions are cations (positively charged ions), such as sodium and potassium, and anions (negatively charged ions), chloride and bicarbonate The AG is the unmeasured anions in a serum sample. The following are examples of these anions:

- Sulfate
- Phosphate
- Lactate
- Pyruvate
- Ketoacids
- Some plasma proteins/amino acids
- Some toxins or toxin metabolites

The normal AG is generally measured at 8–25 mmol/L. An elevated high anion gap (>35) in the metabolic acidosis patient suggests an addition of an unmeasured charged ion producing the acidosis. The following are examples of some of these unmeasured ions:

- Ketoacidosis (diabetes mellitus)
- Hypoadrenocorticism (Addison's disease)
- Lactic acidosis
- Uremia (retention of anion metabolites)
- Toxins (ethylene glycol, methanol, ethanol, paraldehyde (snail bait), aspirin)
- Renal disease

A patient with normal anion gap metabolic acidosis is less common in veterinary medicine and usually associated with increased chloride (**hyperchloremia**). This is generally caused by diseases that produce severe diarrhea and electrolyte abnormalities.

Step 4: Formulate a Treatment Plan

With a patient suffering from respiratory acidosis, when the respiratory acidosis is confirmed by increasing levels of pCO_2 and decreasing pH below normal, the goal to treatment is increasing oxygenation levels. Acute elevations in CO_2 that are due to the anesthetic process require an adjustment of ventilator settings, or manually ventilating the patient. With chronic pulmonary patients, the goal is to increase oxygen levels in the tissue. The overall goals of treatment are the following:

- **On a ventilator:** As with any anesthetic concern, the first step in treating a patient is to increase oxygen concentration and decrease anesthetic levels. Then the goal is to increase oxygen exchange at the alveolar level by decreasing the expiratory time on the ventilator. This produces a deep holding breath that forces gas exchange into the tissue.
- **Without a ventilator:** As stated previously, oxygen concentration should be increased and anesthetic levels decreased. Then the animal should be manually ventilated taking deep breaths until the patient's increased shallow

ventilation slows or blood gases improve. With manual ventilation, the goal is to increase ventilation rate to 15–20 breaths per minute at a pressure of 18–20 cm Hg. **In between each breath, the stop-off valve should be opened to allow the patient to continue breathing on its own and to allow waste gases can be expelled.**

- **With pneumonia patients:** Aggressive therapy is recommended with patients suffering from an infectious disease obstructing alveoli and bronchi and decreasing the body's ability to oxygenate its tissues. Some therapeutic options may be hospitalization, intravenous fluids and antibiotics, oxygen therapy, and nebulization.

With a patient suffering from metabolic acidosis, the key is to treat the primary underlying disease. Through serial blood gas, response to treatment can be evaluated and can be a strong prognostic indicator for the patient's health status. However, in patients that do not respond to standard treatment, bicarbonate therapy may be considered.

To evaluate whether bicarbonate therapy is indicated, base excess (BE) should be evaluated. Base excess indicates the amount of blood buffer available to return blood pH back from acidic level. **If BE is normal in an acidotic patient, there is no need to correct for a metabolic problem.** Base excess is reported in positive or negative numbers.

When faced with a nonresponsive metabolic acidosis with a pH of <7.25, the patient may require intervention other than bolusing a pH balanced fluid. Bicarbonate is dosed according to the following equation:

Sodium bicarbonate (mEq) needed to bring BE to zero = ABS [(weight in kg $\times$ 0.3)

$$\times \text{ BE}]$$

Absolute value (ABS) is needed in this equation or else the value comes back to negative. There is no way to administer a negative amount of bicarbonate.

The medical team must carefully monitor the patient while bicarbonate is given. Generally it is recommended to give half the calculated amount over 30 minutes and reassess acid/base status. Bicarbonate administration should be used cautiously by an experienced medical team.

Last, it is important that the client understands the importance of monitoring blood gas and importance of controlling the acidotic patient. When discussing monitoring blood gas, the medical team should emphasize the following concerns:

- The body requires millions of metabolic reactions to maintain normal function, fight off infection, and deal with disease.
- In order to produce these necessary body reactions, the body must have a blood pH between 7.35–7.45.
- If the blood pH falls below 7.35, the patient becomes acidotic, slowing the body's ability to maintain its normal chemical reactions and adding to the patient's potential for illness and disease.
- One cause of acidosis is respiratory acidosis caused by an inability of the body to exchange gases in the lungs. This is typically seen with patients undergoing long anesthetic procedures, ill patients requiring surgery, and patients with pneumonia.
- The second form of acidosis is metabolic acidosis, which occurs in sick animals that have increased blood or infectious toxin loads, decreased ability to remove toxins from the body (for example, kidney disease, severe dehydration, and other causes), or loss of buffers (from vomiting and diarrhea) that help maintain normal blood pH.
- By evaluating blood gas, the medical team can identify acidotic patients and the type of the acidosis, help identify causes of the acidosis, and identify treatment options that can help stabilize the patient and improve its ability to handle anesthesia or combat severe disease.

13

Coagulation

The bleeding patient can present with acute disease such a hemorrhagic shock or chronic disease causing iron deficiency anemia. In addition, an inability to control the formation of a clot can result in the inappropriate formation of clots (**thrombi**) without injury to a blood vessel. An understanding of the events involved in maintaining adequate blood flow without blood loss is very important when both monitoring a patient's status and relating the results of clinical testing to the condition of the patient. The clinical manifestations of abnormalities in coagulation can assist in determining which of the events in coagulation are dysfunctional. The process of coagulation and the events that control coagulation are complex. This chapter discusses the process of coagulation and the essential steps as they relate to the patient and to laboratory testing.

Blood coagulation (**hemostasis**) is the process of turning free-flowing blood into a stationary clot. This process is essential to life. It prevents fatal blood loss when a vessel or vessels are injured. On the other hand, excessive blood coagulation will result in the formation of blood clots, causing an obstruction of vessels and resulting in hypoxic injury to the tissues. **Fibrinolysis** (breakdown of blood clots) is the opposing mechanism that reestablishes blood flow after the vessel is repaired by dissolving the clot that is obstructing the vessel. Fibrinolysis also limits the process of coagulation to the site of injury. There are several principle events that are involved in coagulation:

- Constriction of the injured vessel
- Formation of the "primary platelet plug"
- Stabilization of the primary platelet plug by deposits of fibrin

Each of these steps is discussed along with the concurrent activation of fibrinolysis as a control of clot formation. Clinical findings and diagnostic testing for disorders of coagulation are reviewed as they relate to the process of hemostasis.

Hemostasis

The three primary elements of hemostasis are the endothelial cells that line the wall of the blood vessels, platelets, and clotting factors. Each of these elements must function appropriately for normal hemostasis. Defects in any of these three participants in the process can result in abnormal bleeding or inappropriate clot formation. Although the processes of hemostasis occur simultaneously in the animal, when a patient is being evaluated for a defect in hemostasis, these processes are considered and tested separately. The most difficult element of hemostasis to evaluate is the endothelial cells.

Endothelial Cells

Endothelial cells line all blood vessels. When injured, the endothelial cell retracts to expose proteins present in the tissue in the vessel wall or interstitium that interact with platelets to promote their adhesion. Further, these sites release molecules that promote activation of the clotting factors. The blood vessel wall plays a major role in both coagulation and fibrinolysis. Interestingly, intact endothelial cells suppress activation of clotting factors and inhibit adhesion of platelets. The dual nature of the endothelial cell assists in keeping the process of coagulation limited to the site of vessel injury.

The intact healthy endothelium has anticoagulant activity. The endothelial cells secrete products that inhibit platelet aggregation (**prostaglandin I and nitrous oxide**), promote vasodilation to keep blood flowing quickly through the lumen, activate anticoagulant proteins (protein C), and promote inactivation of all clotting factors. This anticoagulant activity keeps inappropriate coagulation from occurring in the uninjured vessel. It is extremely important to limit the

process of coagulation to the site of vessel injury. Without this control, the clot would continue to grow and, potentially, block the vessel far beyond what is needed to keep normal blood flow through the vessel.

The injured endothelial cell is procoagulant. The initial action of the endothelial cell is to contract and constrict the vessel. This immediate action decreases the flow of blood. The injured endothelial cells expose subendothelial tissues that activate platelets and promote their aggregation. In addition, the injured endothelial cells bind clotting factors on their surface, which increases their concentration at the site of injury. At the same time, injured endothelial cells release proteins that oppose fibrinolysis. The focal inhibition of fibrinolysis allows the developing clot to be strong.

There is no laboratory testing that can evaluate the function of endothelial cells. There are diseases that can interfere with the function of the endothelial cells. In most cases, abnormal endothelial cells result in abnormal clot formation because they do not maintain their anticoagulant nature. Sepsis and metabolic diseases such as diabetes can result in procoagulant changes in endothelial cells throughout the body.

Platelets

Platelets are essential for primary hemostasis, the formation of the initial clot (primary platelet plug). The injured endothelial cells promote the adhesion, aggregation, swelling, and secretion by platelets (activation). Activated platelets also promote the activation of other platelets. Platelets are very sensitive to endothelial cell injury, which is why it is important to perform atraumatic venipuncture. Any trauma to the vessel or surrounding tissue during venipuncture will activate platelets and result in platelet clumping in the blood sample. When platelets are activated, they release factors that promote activation of the coagulation cascade. In addition to the secreted factors, platelets provide a surface for the clotting process and the cellular mass that will form the clot.

Defects in primary hemostasis can occur due to decreased numbers of circulating platelets (**thrombocytopenia**) or platelet dysfunction. **Thrombocytopenia is the most common defect in primary hemostasis.** Thrombocytopenia can be due to several mechanisms, as discussed in Chapter 4. Defects in platelet function, most often hereditary, include the following:

- Deficiencies in factors that allow the platelet to adhere to the subendothelial tissue, as seen in **von Willebrand's disease** (e.g., Doberman Pinscher)
- Factors that allow platelets to adhere to each other, as seen in **Glanzmann's thrombasthenia** (e.g., Great Pyrenees)
- Factors that allow the platelet to adhere to von Willebrand's factor as seen in **Bernard-Soulier syndrome**

In addition, there are inherited diseases that affect the contents of the granules in the platelet that inhibit release of procoagulant factors. There are acquired defects in platelet function; the most common is drug related. Aspirin and certain antiinflammatory drugs inhibit platelet function.

Thrombocytopenia or platelet dysfunction produce an overt "primary" hemorrhage, petechia and hemorrhage from mucosal surfaces (melena, epistaxis).

Coagulation Factors

Secondary hemostasis is the process of stabilizing the platelet plug by formation of **fibrin**, the mortar that holds the platelets together. Again, in the patient, the processes of primary and secondary hemostasis occur simultaneously. The formation of stable fibrin is the result of activation of numerous circulating clotting factors that are enzymes or enzyme complexes that form the coagulation cascade. The coagulation cascade depends on many cofactors, such as calcium and multiple feedback loops that accelerate and inhibit the process. If there is a deficiency in the coagulation cascade, the primary plug will degrade prematurely and bleeding will resume.

For the purpose of discussion, the coagulation cascade (the sequential steps involved in clotting) are artificially separated into two pathways that converge into a common pathway that ends in the formation of fibrin. **Fibrinogen** is the protein precursor to fibrin that circulates in the plasma. In the coagulation cascade, the two pathways are the **intrinsic pathway**, where all the factors are found in the blood, and the **extrinsic pathway**, which requires a tissue factor. Figure 13.1 illustrates the two converging pathways and the final pathway. It is very important to remember that this separation of pathways is artificial. In the animal, it is easier to think of the intrinsic pathway as an acceleration pathway that amplifies the extrinsic pathway. The central theme for the coagulation cascade is to form fibrin, and the major factor involved in formation of fibrin is the enzyme **thrombin**. One could say that the formation of thrombin and control of its activity is the primary purpose of the coagulation cascade.

Thrombin is a powerful enzyme that circulates in the blood in an inactive form called **prothrombin**. Thrombin converts the circulating protein fibrinogen into fibrin, the glue that holds the platelet plug together (Figure 13.2). However, transforming fibrinogen into fibrin is not the only process in which thrombin plays a role. Thrombin promotes platelet aggregation, activates several clotting factors, and inhibits the breakdown of fibrin. In addition, thrombin also plays a role in inhibiting coagulation. Thrombin activates a molecule that inhibits its own actions. Where it is in high concentration (in the area where the clot is

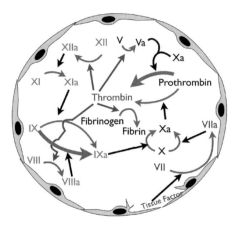

Figure 13.1. The intrinsic pathway is green, the extrinsic pathway is blue, and the common pathway is in black. The figure illustrates the interaction of the three pathways with feedback loops to amplify the production of thrombin. The thrombin produced then amplifies the intrinsic and common pathway.

forming), thrombin will degrade activated clotting factors.

Defects in secondary hemostasis can be acquired or inherited. Inherited disorders of coagulation occur when the patient cannot produce a specific clotting factor or produces an abnormal, inactive clotting factor. The most common clotting factor deficiencies are

- Hemophilia A (deficiency of factor VIII)
- Hemophilia B (deficiency of factor IX)
- Deficiency of factor X

Acquired disorders of coagulation are diseases that result in decreased production of clotting factors from liver failure (see Chapter 6), increased consumption of clotting factors (disseminated intravascular coagulation), or ingestion of toxins that inhibit the function of clotting factors (warfarin toxicity).

Factors that evaluate liver damage and dysfunction have been discussed in Chapter 6. Patients with increased liver dysfunction can have decreased production of clotting factors, which can make them more prone to bleed. Medical teams evaluating patients for suspected liver disease and failure should not draw blood from large veins (e.g., the jugular vein) because this may produce serious bleeding into the tissue.

Warfarin toxicity is one of the more common acquired coagulation disorders. Warfarin is a toxin that acts as a vitamin K antagonist. Vitamin K is extremely important in the production of functional coagulation factors. Vitamin K is a cofactor that is necessary for a specific enzyme used in producing clotting factors II, VII, IX, X and the anticoagulant factors protein C and S.

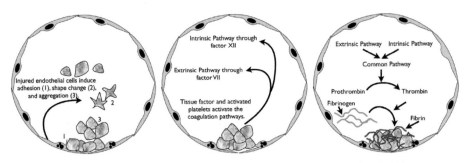

Figure 13.2. Damage to the endothelial cells exposes receptors (von Willebrand factor) and platelets adhere to the wall of the vessel covering the defect. The platelets become activated, undergo a shape change, and begin to aggregate to form a clot at the injury. The platelets secrete substances and provide tissue factor for activation of the clotting factors. Once the coagulation pathways are activated, prothrombin is converted to thrombin, thrombin converts fibrinogen to fibrin, and the fibrin "glues" the platelets together into a stable clot sealing off the injury.

Disseminated intravascular coagulation (DIC) is a syndrome that is seen in association with many disease processes. Any disease that results in a procoagulation state can initiate DIC. Systemic activation of platelets and the coagulation cascade causes the formation of small clots (**microthrombi**) throughout the capillaries of the vascular system and consumption of both platelets and clotting factors. Simultaneously, the fibrinolytic system is activated. Early in the process, the individual will be hypercoagulable, and as the process progresses and platelets and coagulation factors are depleted, uncontrolled bleeding occurs. The condition is best treated by addressing the underlying disease. Common diseases associated with DIC include heat stroke, endotoxemia (sepsis), severe trauma, shock, neoplasia, venomous bites, and vasculitis. The results of DIC can be seen on the blood film in the form of red cell fragments (**schistocytes**, see Chapter 3) and decreased platelet numbers. The microthrombi can result in multiple organ failure.

Disseminated intravascular coagulation, widespread activation of the coagulation factors, results in formation of small microclots that obstruction flow through capillary beds. This in turn leads to consumption of platelets in the microthrombi resulting in thrombocytopenia. **Coagulation tests become prolonged when 75% of the coagulation factors are absent.** Decreased production of clotting factors by the liver occurs when 75% of functional liver mass is lost. The prothrombin time (PT) and activated partial thromboplastin time (APTT) are the most common coagulation tests done in practice. These tests are performed most often at a reference laboratory.

Fibrinolysis

Hemostasis is the process of clotting, and fibrinolysis is the process of dissolution of a clot. Both of these processes are complex and closely intertwined. They occur almost simultaneously with coagulation limited to the site of vessel injury and fibrinolysis at the edge of the developing clot to localize the process of coagulation to the injury. Eventually, once the vessel is repaired, fibrinolysis removes the clot and blood flow through the injured vessel is reestablished. There are rare inherited disorders of fibrinolysis that can result in an increased tendency to form clots (thrombosis).

Diagnostic Tests for Coagulation Abnormalities

The tests used to identify the cause of bleeding are separated into those that address primary hemostasis (platelet numbers and function) and those used to evaluate secondary hemostasis (clotting factors). The most important aspect of testing for abnormalities in hemostasis is sample collection.

Primary Hemostasis

The platelet count is the most common test for defects in primary hemostasis. **In general, an animal will not begin to spontaneously bleed until the platelet number is <40,000/μL.** An EDTA tube is used for determination of platelet numbers. It is essential that the venipuncture is as atraumatic as possible to decrease the activation of platelets. In addition, for optimum evaluation of the platelet count, the count should be performed within 4 hours of collection. As discussed in Chapter 2, platelet numbers can be estimated from the blood film as well.

Platelet function tests should be performed in the bleeding patient with normal platelet numbers and coagulation times. There are sensitive tests for platelet

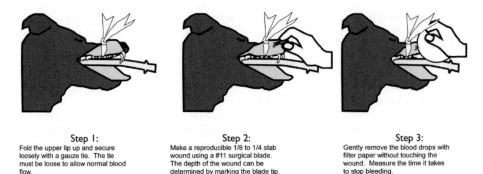

Step 1:
Fold the upper lip up and secure loosely with a gauze tie. The tie must be loose to allow normal blood flow.

Step 2:
Make a reproducible 1/8 to 1/4 stab wound using a #11 surgical blade. The depth of the wound can be determined by marking the blade tip.

Step 3:
Gently remove the blood drops with filter paper without touching the wound. Measure the time it takes to stop bleeding.

Figure 13.3. A method for determining the buccal mucosal bleeding time.

function that require submission of a sample to a specialty laboratory. However, there are in-house tests that can be done to identify patients with possible defects in platelet function: **buccal mucosal bleeding time, cuticle bleeding time, and clot retraction.** The cuticle bleeding time and clot retraction tests are very insensitive and are not recommended. The cuticle bleeding time will be prolonged with defects in coagulation as well as decreased platelet function. The clot retraction test (measuring the time from collection to complete retraction of the clot and separation of serum) requires normal platelet numbers and normal function. The maximum time for normal retraction of the clot is 1–2 hours.

The **buccal mucosal bleeding** time is commonly done to screen dogs for von Willebrand's disease. A small shallow cut is made in the mucosal surface of the upper lip, and the time from the initial cut to cessation of bleeding is recorded. It is very important to perform this test in a standard and consistent manner. A standard procedure for this test is outlined in Figure 13.3. If there is a prolonged buccal mucosal bleeding time, further laboratory tests are required to determine the cause of the platelet dysfunction.

Secondary Hemostasis

The common tests for defects in secondary hemostasis are the **prothrombin time (PT)** and the **activated partial thromboplastin time (aPTT).** The PT assay evaluates the extrinsic pathway and the aPTT assay evaluates the intrinsic pathway.

When drawing blood for coagulation time testing, the quality of the sample plays a major part in providing accurate results. The volume collected in the vacutainer is critical. Using the vacutainer sleeve is the best way to insure proper filling of the vacutainer with minimum hemolysis and activation of platelets. To obtain the best possible sample, place a catheter for collection. Before drawing the sample into the citrate tube (blue top), clear the catheter needle and tubing by drawing a small amount of blood into a serum tube (red top); then allow the citrate tube to fill completely.

When using a syringe and needle, it is essential to perform an atraumatic venipuncture. If possible, change syringes after drawing 0.5 mL of blood to clear the needle of any tissue or activated platelets. Immediately transfer the correct amount of blood to the collection tube. You can transfer the blood using the vacuum of the collection

tube. If the collection tube is over- or underfilled, the results of the coagulation tests
will be affected.

It is optimum to perform coagulation
tests within 4 hours of collection. If using
a reference laboratory with a local courier,
centrifuge and separate the plasma from the
cells immediately using a plastic pipette to
transfer the plasma to a clean plastic tube.
Keep the sample cold until picked up by
the laboratory courier. If using a reference
laboratory by overnight delivery, freeze at
$-20°C$ or lower if testing will be delayed
for more than 24 hours. Ship the sample
overnight with cold packs or dry ice. Multiple freezing and thawing can artifactually

Table 13.1. Causes of prolonged clotting times.

Primary hemostasis		
Test	Outcome	
Platelet count	Decreased platelet number will affect the body's ability to produce the initial clot (<40,000/µL).	
Platelet function tests	Sent out to lab when presented with a bleeding animal with normal platelet number and normal clotting times.	
Buccal mucosal bleeding	Done as an in-house test for lack of von Willebrand's factor (von Willebrand's disease)	

Secondary hemostasis		
Test	Cascade Affected	Possible Causes
Prolonged PT Normal aPTT	Extrinsic cascade	Factor VII deficiency
Normal PT Prolonged aPTT	Intrinsic cascade	Factor VIII or IX deficiency
Prolonged PT Prolonged aPTT	Both cascades	Multiple factor deficiencies • Vitamin K antagonism (rat poison) • Liver disease • DIC Inherited Dz: • Factor X • Thrombin

prolong coagulation tests. Plasma from a healthy dog can be sent with the patient's sample as a control.

Although clotting times can vary from lab to lab, normal levels are generally as seen in Charts 13.1 and 13.2.

Chart 13.1 Prothrombin Times (PT)—Measurement of the Extrinsic Pathway

Canine	12–17 sec
Feline	15–23 sec

Chart 13.2 Partial Prothrombin Times (aPTT)—Measurement of the Intrinsic Pathway

Canine	71–102 sec
Feline	70–120 sec

Both tests are performed for a full evaluation of the coagulation cascade. A prolonged PT and normal aPTT indicate defect in the extrinsic pathway (usually a deficiency in factor VII); a prolonged aPTT with a normal PT indicate a defect in the extrinsic pathway (usually a defect in either factor IX or VIII). If both tests are prolonged, there may be multiple factor deficiencies (vitamin K antagonism or warfarin toxicity, liver disease, DIC) or an inherited defect in factor X or thrombin).

Another test is the **whole blood clotting time**, which is a measure of the time it takes for blood drawn into a serum tube to clot. In the normal dog, the blood should clot within 3–15 min, in the cat, 6–8 min. This is a crude measure of secondary hemostasis. If prolonged it indicates severe multiple factor deficiency such as warfarin toxicity, severe liver disease, or DIC.

Finally, there are tests that are used primarily for evaluation of the patient suspected of having DIC. In addition to clotting times and platelet counts, tests that identify increased degradation of fibrin can be performed. **Fibrinogen degradation product (FDP)** and **D-dimer assays** both identify fragments of fibrin that occur with excessive fibrinolysis. Both of these tests are best performed at a reference laboratory. However, since DIC is a life-threatening condition that must be treated quickly, medical teams do not usually have the time to wait for outside lab analysis to be completed (Table 13.1). Therefore, both the FDP and D-dimer assays are more often confirmatory tests rather than diagnostic tests.

Emergency Diagnostics—A Discussion of Shock and Clinical Diagnostics

Obtaining a clinical diagnostics baseline in the emergency patient can vary dependent on how the patient presents, the chief complaint, and the needs of the medical team. However, when faced with an emergency patient a minimal clinical database can be obtained. There are different levels of clinical diagnostics that can be obtained. The following levels of clinical diagnostics can suggest a testing hierarchy.

Code I Database

A code I database is obtained as an initial diagnostic baseline for the emergency patient. The information is obtained quickly from a very small sample of blood (i.e., with a catheter stilette) and a quick evaluation of monitoring modalities. Although not a full clinical diagnostic, careful attention to changes in a code I database can help

the medical teams quickly create an effective problem list (Table 14.1).

Obtaining Blood Samples

The most effective way of obtaining diagnostic samples from the emergency patient is to fill the blood tubes through a nonheparinized/nonflushed peripheral catheter that is being set prior to the administration of fluids. In some cases, where patients are very hypotensive, obtaining adequate samples is not possible. If blood has to be drawn from another source, it is recommended to obtain a sample from a small peripheral vein until clotting times can be evaluated. On initial blood collection, the blood tubes should always be checked for abnormalities that can suggest serious disease or pathology (see Chapters 1 and 2). The following sections review recommended clinical diagnostics.

Table 14.1.   An overview of code I diagnostics.

Clinical Test	Outcome	Other Diagnostics	Cause/Action
Packed cell volume	Canine >55% Feline >45 %	Should be a marked increase in albumin/total protein.	Dehydration 1. Notify veterinarian. 2. Prepare patient for aggressive fluid therapy.
	Canine <35 % Feline <25 %	Check purple top for clot or agglutination. Check albumin/total protein for decrease. Check a blood film for abnormal cellularity (i.e. spherocytes).	**Notify veterinarian.** Causes: • Blood loss • Chronic anemia of disease • IMHA • Artifact
Serum	Straw-colored	If hemolyzed, check PCV for anemia; check purple top for agglutination. If icteric, check PCV for anemia and purple top for agglutination. Check patient for physical jaundice. If lipemic, check medical history for the last time patient ate.	Document all changes to serum and notify veterinarian.
Buffy coat	Buffy coat should be <1% but visible	Check white blood cell count and blood film.	Decreased buffy coat: viral infection/immunosuppression Increased buffy coat: infection/inflammation/cancer
Total protein	Canine: 5–7.2 g/dL Feline: 5.8–8.5 g/dL	Low total protein: Evaluate PCV/TP, albumin. High total protein: Evaluate PCV/TP, albumin and globulin.	Low total protein can suggest bleeding, renal disease, liver disease, chronic intestinal disease, or possibly disease that produces a decreased immune response (low immunoglobulin). High total protein: dehydration or disease that produces an increased immune response (high immunoglobulin)
Albumin	Canine: 3.1–4.5 g/dL Feline: 2.4–4.1 g/dL	Low albumin: Evaluate PCV/TP, clotting times, urinalysis, renal enzymes, liver enzymes. High albumin: Evaluate PCV/TP.	Low total protein can suggest bleeding, renal disease, liver disease, chronic intestinal disease. High total protein: dehydration
Blood glucose	Canine: 60–115 mg/dL Feline: 60–130 mg/dL	Low blood glucose: Check white blood cell count/blood film. Increased blood glucose: urinalysis, fructosamine, chemistry	Low blood sugar: sepsis **Notify veterinarian immediately.** Increased blood glucose: diabetes mellitus, stress

Table 14.1.   *(Continued)*

Clinical Test	Outcome	Other Diagnostics	Cause/Action
Electrolytes	Sodium (Na): Canine: 142–150 mEq/L Feline: 147–162 mEq/L Chloride (Cl): Canine: 105–117 mEq/L Feline: 114–126 mEq/L Potassium (K): Canine: 4.5–5.4 mEq/L Feline: 3.7–5.2 mEq/L	Chemistry Urinalysis	Decrease in electrolytes is caused by vomiting, diarrhea, fluid therapy. Increase in potassium: FLUTD, hypoadrenocorticism **Notify veterinarian immediately.**
Lactate	Lactate >3 (Although normal can vary from machine to machine.)	Blood gas	Increased lactate supports decreased ability to oxygenate tissue (perfusion). This makes the tissue burn energy through fermentation and lactate builds up. Serial lactates serve as a monitor of how the body is responding to treatment to increase oxygenation of blood and body perfusion.
Clotting times	PT: Canine: 71–102 sec Feline 70–120 sec aPTT: Canine: 12–17 sec Feline: 15–23 sec	Increased clotting times: Evaluate PCV/ TP, Albumin, CBC (platelet count)	Increased clotting times support the patient's ability to clot blood (see Chapter). **Notify veterinarian immediately.**
Blood pressure	Systolic >100–140 mm Hg		If there are any abnormalities, **notify veterinarian immediately.**

Packed Cell Volume (PCV)/Total Protein (TP)

A PCV/TP is one of the first tests that should be completed on an emergency patient (Figure 14.1). The PCV/TP should be evaluated for serum color, red blood cell concentration, buffy coat, and total protein levels.

Step 1: Evaluate and Record Serum Color

Normal serum should be straw-colored or clear. Changes in serum color can indicate disease or artifact. Changes in serum color should be documented in the chart and discussed with the veterinarian, because serum changes can affect chemistry results in hospital machinery. The following sections review serum abnormalities.

Red

Red coloration of the serum can artifactually elevate kidney, liver, and electrolyte levels on some in house chemistry equipment. The red coloration can occur with artifact or disease.

Artifact: Traumatic blood stick or collection

Packed Cell Volume
or Hematocrit

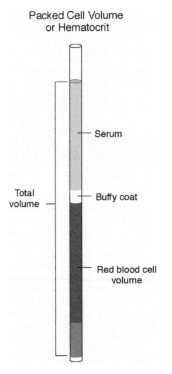

Figure 14.1. Illustration of a PCV tube with the separation of red blood cells, buffy coat (white blood cells), and serum.

Disease: Hemolysis of red blood cells occurs within the vessels because white blood cells are destroying red blood cells as if they were foreign bacteria. This change is secondary to an immune-mediated hemolytic anemia (IMHA).

White

White coloration suggests an accumulation of fat within the serum or fluid portion of the blood. It can have effect on several parameters in the chemistry and also can occur with artifact or disease.

Artifact: Pets that have eaten within a few hours of blood draw may have a postprandial increased fat level.

Disease: Increased lipemia can occur with diseases that alter fat digestion. The following are some examples of these diseases:

- Hypothyroidism
- Diabetes mellitus
- Hyperadrenocorticism (Cushing's disease)
- Hyperlipidemia

Yellow

A yellow pigmentation (**jaundice**) suggests a buildup of toxin from the inability of the liver to detoxify, a massive destruction of red blood cells in the vessels, or a gallbladder obstruction. Jaundice always suggests one of the following diseases:

- Liver disease
- Immune-mediated hemolytic anemia
- Gallbladder disease

Step 2: Evaluate the Packed Cell Volume (PCV) Percentage

The next step is to evaluate the red blood cell column as compared to the entire column of blood and fluid. This is called the packed cell volume percentage.

Normal PCV

Chart 14.1 lists normal PCV percentages.

Chart 14.1

Canine	35–55%
Feline	25–45%

Decreased PCV

Decreased PCV can indicate dilution, blood clot, or anemia:

- **Dilution:** If too little blood is placed in a purple top tube, the blood will be diluted by the EDTA in the tube, lowering the packed cell volume. If there is only a small sample available, micro blood tubes are available from your lab. These tubes require only 250–500 µL of blood.

- **Blood clot:** If the blood is not adequately mixed with the EDTA, the blood may clot, artifactually lowering the packed cell volume.
- **Anemia:** Anemia or a decreased red blood cell count can be caused by
  - **Blood loss/internal bleeding:** Acute blood loss or internal bleeding can lower PCV. When the patient acutely bleeds, both PCV and TP decrease as protein follows blood out of the vascular supply. **Team members should check total protein/albumin to help determine whether the anemia is caused by blood loss.**
  - **Chronic anemia of disease:** Chronic disease that decreases the body's ability to regenerate red blood cells can produce a severe anemia. Diseases that can produce chronic anemia are kidney disease, liver disease, or cancer.
  - **Immune-mediated hemolytic anemia:** As discussed previously, destruction of the red blood cells by white blood cells, as if they were foreign bacteria, can also cause severe anemia. **Team members should evaluate the purple top tube and blood film for agglutination or the presence of spherocytes on the blood film.**

Increased PCV

Increased PCV generally suggests **dehydration**. With a dehydrated patient, the fluid component of the blood decreases, increasing the overall percentage of red cells compared to the column of blood.

Step 3: Check the Buffy Coat

Dramatic changes in the buffy coat can suggest increases in the white blood cell count secondary to infection, inflammation, or—rarely—neoplasia. If the white blood cell count elevates, discuss running a CBC to the lab to help quantitate the total white blood cell count and the types of white blood cells elevating.

Step 4: Evaluate Total Protein/Albumin

Total protein is the sum of two body proteins: globulin produced by the lymphocytes to fight off infection, and albumin produced by the liver to carry other chemicals throughout the bloodstream. Dehydration, blood loss, and organ disease can effect albumin and thus affect total protein levels. Normal total protein and normal albumin levels are listed in Charts 14.2 and 14.3, respectively.

Chart 14.2   Total Protein

Canine	5.0–7.2 g/dL
Feline	5.8–8.5 g/dL

Chart 14.3   Albumin

Canine	3.1–4.5 g/dL
Feline	2.4–4.1 g/dL

Decreased Total Protein/Albumin Levels

Decreased levels of albumin can occur with severe blood loss or organ disease.

With bleeding, albumin follows blood out through the vessels lowering body albumin levels. However, diseases that affect the excretion (loss), production, or absorption of protein can also cause a low body albumin level. Further, albumin maintains a positive pressure (oncotic pressure) on fluid components within blood. When albumin levels decrease, this pressure is lost and fluid more readily flows into surrounding tissue.

Low albumin levels can make a patient more at risk for fluid overload and pulmonary edema.

Increased Total Protein/Albumin Levels

Similar to the packed cell volume, as an animal dehydrates, albumin concentrates in the decreased blood fluid, increasing their measurable levels.

Blood Film

As discussed in Chapter 3, a thorough blood film should be completed with a full complete blood count, and blood film review is part of a code II database. However a brief review of blood films while obtaining a code I database can be extremely benefi-cial in evaluating the patient's overall condition. Although discussed previously, the blood film should be evaluated for the following parameters (Figures 14.2, 14.3).

Low-Power Review of Blood Film (10×)

A precursory qualitative evaluation should be done to determine the number of white blood cells and if microfilaria or giant cells are present (see Chapter 4).

High-Power Review of Blood Film (100×, Oil Immersion)

The following parameters should be evaluated and documented for n a brief review of the blood film.

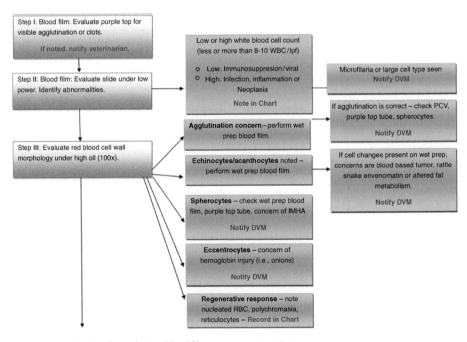

Figure 14.2. Algorithm for evaluating blood film on emergency patients.

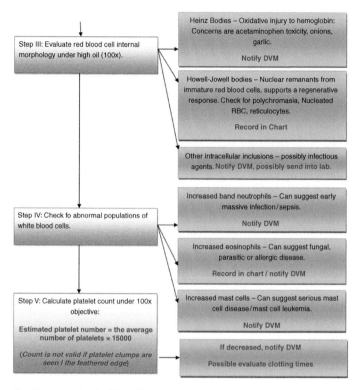

Figure 14.3. Algorithm for evaluating blood film on emergency patients.

Red Blood Cell Morphology

Red blood cells should be evaluated for the following changes suggestive of disease pathology:

- Changes in the lipid membrane:
  - Agglutination
  - Spherocytes
  - Acanthocytes/echinocytes
  - Schistocytes
  - Nucleated red blood cells/poly-chromasia
- Changes in the red blood cell internal morphology:
  - Heinz bodies
  - Howell-Jolly Body
  - Other intracellular changes (i.e., Infectious agents)

White Blood Cells

White blood cells should be evaluated for the following changes:

- Increased band neutrophils
- Increased eosinophils
- Mast cell present

Platelet Estimate

The platelet estimate should be evaluated.

Blood Sugar

Blood sugar levels should be monitored regularly and should always be obtained from all critical care animals on presentation. Normal glucose levels are listed in Chart 14.4.

Chart 14.4

Canine	60–125 mg/dL
Feline	70–150 mg/dL

An animal can show severe weakness or neurologic signs and it may simply be attributable to a low blood sugar.

Low blood sugar levels (<50 mg/dL) can produce the following:

- Seizures
- Weakness
- Collapse
- Anorexia
- Ataxia
- Abnormal vocalization
- Coma
- Death

Using a Human Glucometer

This is extremely helpful in obtaining a quick glucose level with very little blood. However, human glucometers are adjusted low (40–50 mg/dL glucose) to encourage human diabetics to eat before glucose drops too low. **Remember 60–80 mg/dL glucose on a glucometer may be 100–110 mg/dL to the animal.**

Electrolytes

Electrolytes refer to sodium, potassium, and chloride (see Chapter 8). These minerals are responsible for normal fluid balance in the body, conduction of nerve impulses, muscular contraction, and concentration of urine. **As discussed previously normal sodium,** chloride, and potassium levels are listed in Charts 14.5, 14.6, and 14.7, respectively.

Chart 14.5   Sodium (Na)

Canine	142–150 mEq/L
Feline	147–162 mEq/L

Chart 14.6   Chloride (Cl)

Canine	105–117 mEq/L
Feline	114–126 mEq/L

Chart 14.7   Potassium (K)

Canine	4.0–5.4 mEq/L
Feline	3.7–5.2 mEq/L

Animals with severe derangement of electrolytes can show serious to life-threatening signs:

- Slow heart rate
- Pulse deficits
- Muscle fasciculations (muscle tremors/shaking)
- Weakness
- Anorexia

Animals that are on long-term fluids (>24 hours) and not eating and drinking can also have severe aberrations of electrolytes in the body. Most animals that have vomiting or diarrhea can have severe electrolyte changes. These electrolytes can be added or balanced dependent on blood electrolyte levels.

Clotting Times

If there are concerns of increased chances of bleeding, routine clotting times may be needed (see Chapter 13). Normal values are listed in Chart 14.8.

Chart 14.8

Test	Canine	Feline
APTT	71–102 sec	70–120 sec
PT	12–17 sec	15–23 sec

Any animals with severe metabolic derangements and disease can begin to have problems with their ability to clot. The following are some types of diseases that cause clotting problems:

- GDV/bloat
- Splenectomy
- Liver disease (severe)
- Heat stroke
- Pancreatitis (severe)
- Types of cancer
- Massive infection (sepsis)

Lactate

As a patient has decreased ability to perfuse tissue, conversion of glucose into carbon dioxide and energy in the cellular level is also decreased. Decreased oxygen tension at the cellular level makes the body use fermentation to produce energy. This less efficient pathway builds up lactate as a byproduct; increased presence of this acid can cause the patient to have metabolic acidosis. Increased body lactate represents a medical concern and supports a patient's inability to perfuse tissue. A patient under treatment with lactate levels that return to normal suggests that perfusion is improving. Normal Values are listed in Chart 14.9.

Chart 14.9

Test	Canine	Feline
Lactate	<3 sec	<3 sec

Lactate should be evaluated in animals that are unable to perfuse and oxygenate their tissues (e.g., cardiac disease, pulmonary disease [pneumonia]) to assess how severe decreased oxygenation is affecting the tissue. Higher levels of lactate suggest more severe concern to oxygenate and perfuse the body. As the animal is treated, decreasing lactate levels can suggest a response to treatment. Further, patients that may have vascular compromise to their tissues (e.g., gastro-distention volvulus), lactate levels can suggest how much tissue damage due to lack of oxygenation (**ischemia**) may be occurring. In these cases, patients with increasing lactate levels may have more tissue damage and death.

Blood Pressure

Systolic blood pressure is a measure of the body's ability to perfuse tissue and organs. In an emergency situation, the hospital team's ability to restore normal perfusion is the key to stabilization and a normal return for organ function (e.g., glomerular filtration, hepatic detoxification). Normal systolic nlood pressure levels are listed in Chart 14.10.

Chart 14.10

Test	Canine	Feline
Systolic blood pressure	100–140 mm HG	100–160 mm HG

Hypotension

Systolic blood pressures <100 mm Hg suggest that the patient in unable to adequately perfuse their tissues and organs. This indicates that the body is unable to filter toxins, produce and transport needed protein and energy sources, and produce an adequate immune response. **Until blood systolic blood pressure is >100 mg Hg, the patient is still unstable.**

Trauma Patients

Trauma patients (e.g., those hit by a car) may initially come in hypotensive, and normal perfusion can be restored with aggressive fluid therapy. However, it is important for team members to monitor blood pressure as patients stabilize so that pressures do not rise to >130–140 mm HG. **Increased pressures above this level may overcome clots that have already formed secondary to internal trauma and may restart internal bleeding.** Once normal blood pressure is restored, trauma patients should have PCV/TP and clotting times reevaluated to determine the risk of internal bleeding.

Hypertension

Hypertension may occur secondary to many chronic disease conditions of middle-aged to older patients. Aggressive fluid therapy can make patients more hypertensive, leading to fluid overload, heart failure, retinal lesions, shock, and death. Diseases that can cause hypertension are renal disease, hyperthyroidism (feline), hyperadrenocorticism (Cushing's disease), heart disease, and primary hypertension.

Code II Database

A code II database is obtained when the patient is stable and undergoing treatment. Sample collection and diagnostic testing may need to be performed based on the patient's comfort and stability level. Code II diagnostics come into play as the animal is stabilized and moved into a critical care nursing phase. Code II databases can include the following:

- Complete blood count
- Thorough blood film analysis
- Chemistry
- Urinalysis
- Full electrolyte profile
- Blood gas
- Radiography
- Ultrasound

Code III Database

A code III database may contain elements of all previous databases, but it is generally obtained on completely stable patients that may be treated in hospital or as outpatients. These databases can include the following:

- Infectious screens
- Thyroid profiles
- Adrenal axis testing
- Endoscopy
- Laparoscopy
- Exploratory surgery
- Advanced Image Scanning: fluoroscopy, MRI, cat scan

Obtaining Samples from Different Body Systems and Evaluating Cytology

Cytology is the study of cellular samples from fluid or tissue prepared directly on glass slides and stained for microscopic evaluation. Cytology is less invasive than tissue biopsies and in some cases can provide a rapid diagnosis that would otherwise take several days if done by histopathology.

The procedure for obtaining a cytological sample is less complicated and, in many cases, can be done without anesthesia. As a result, cytology offers less risk to the patient. There are rare complications associated with fine needle aspiration. Table 15.1 lists possible complications associated with different sites. The primary disadvantage of using cytology for evaluation of a disease process is the fact that only individual cells without any tissue architecture are observed. This is primarily a problem if **neoplasia** (cancer) is a concern. In many cases of potential neoplasia, a follow-up biopsy is needed to confirm the diagnosis. It is important that the client understand the possibility of further testing in these cases.

Common cytological samples include body cavity fluids, tracheal washes, or bronchoalveolar lavage (fluid flushed in and reaspirated through an endotracheal tube or bronchoscope), fine needle aspiration of cutaneous or internal masses (cells drawn into a syringe), imprints of surface lesions and masses removed for biopsy, swabs of surface lesions, and scrapings of skin lesions.

Cytological preparations are usually read by the veterinarian or submitted to a laboratory for evaluation by a veterinary pathologist. The veterinary technician is often responsible for preparing the sample for evaluation by the veterinarian or submission to the laboratory. Technicians may be responsible for performing the initial evaluation of skin scrapings and ear swab preparations.

The quality of the information obtained from any cytological procedure depends greatly on the quality of the preparation itself. Obtaining a high-quality cytological sample requires patience and practice. Artifacts that can interfere with cytological evaluation include the following:

- Too few cells
- Thick preparations

Table 15.1. Complications associated with fine needle aspiration.

Complication	Site
Pneumothorax	Lung
Hemorrhage	Liver, kidney, spleen, lung
Tumor seeding	Neoplastic lesions
Bacteremia	Abscess (internal or external)
Sepsis	Abscess (internal or external)

- Preparations with stain precipitate or ultrasound gel
- Inadequate staining
- Excessive lysis of cells

How a sample is handled prior to microscopic evaluation will have a great impact on the usefulness of the procedure. This chapter provides an overview of cytology, with emphasis on sample collection and preparation of slides for microscopic viewing. A short section on cytological findings is included to familiarize the technician with the types of diseases that lend themselves to a cytological diagnosis.

Types of Cytological Preparations

The most common cytological samples used in veterinary medicine for evaluation of disease processes, in order of frequency of use, are skin scrapings and ear swabs, fine needle aspirates of mass lesion, aspiration of body cavity fluids, and imprints of skin lesions or excised tissue. Skin scrapings and ear swabs are primarily used to identify infectious agents such as **dermatophytic fungi (ringworm)**, mites (***Demodex*** spp, ***Sarcoptes*** spp), yeasts (***Malassezia*** spp) and bacteria (***Staphylococcus*** spp). Scrapings are most commonly evaluated by the veterinarian or technician to assist in determining if infectious disease is the cause of dermatitis (inflammation of the skin) or otitis externa (inflammation of the external ear).

Skin Scrapings

Skin scrapings are usually obtained by aggressively scraping the surface of the skin lesion until it bleeds. It is important to scrape deep enough into the dermis because dermatophytes and mites such as *Demodex* sp. are usually within or around hair follicles. Although some mite species such as *Sarcoptes* spp are superficial, deep scrapings will get both mite species. When evaluating for dermatophytes, a potassium hydroxide solution (5–15% KOH) is often used to dissolve keratin debris in the skin scraping. However, KOH preparations can be difficult to evaluate without significant experience. Figure 15.1 shows photomicrographs of scrapings from a dog with demodecosis and a cat with dermatophytosis.

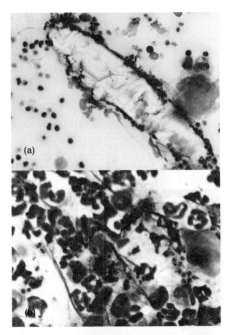

Figure 15.1. (a) *Demodex canis* mite, deep skin scraping from a dog with generalized dermatitis. **(b)** Arthroconidia of *Microsporum canis* (small round blue-staining spores), fine needle aspirate of a skin mass from a dog with a single mass lesion.

Swabs

Culture swabs can be used to obtain cells from a surface lesion, a draining tract, the ear, and the vagina. The samples are prepared by swabbing the site and rolling the swab onto a glass slide. Even though the identification of infectious agents is often a concern with this type of cytology preparation, they do not need any other stain than routine Wright-Giemsa stain used for blood films. Bacteria and fungal elements will stain deeply basophilic (purple). Figure 15.2 shows an ear swab preparation with scattered *Malassezia* sp. yeast elements.

Because skin scrapings and ear swabs often contain bacteria and yeast, it is recommended that a separate set of staining stations be used for these preparations. Several bacteria and yeast organisms can grow in the stain solutions. As a result of this growth, stains used routinely for surface lesions should be changed more often than those used for other types of cytological preparations.

Imprint Preparations

Imprint cytology is probably the least common type of cytological preparation. The

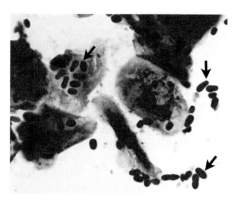

Figure 15.2. *Malessizia* sp., ear swab from a dog.

preparations are made by pressing a glass slide onto a surface lesion or by lightly touching a portion of an excised tissue to the slide. Preparing a good imprint requires patience and a light touch. When sampling a surface lesion, a two-step process provides the most information. The first imprint is made of the lesion before cleaning the site. The second imprint is made after the site is cleaned. If there is the possibility that a culture will be needed, the site should be surgically prepared after the cytological preparations have been made. An imprint preparation of an excised lesion can provide a quick assessment of the lesion. The optimum surface size of tissue for an imprint is less than 1 cm^2. In order to insure the adherence of cells to the slide, it is important to blot all surface fluid from the sample before making the imprint. Once the surface is blotted, the tissue is lightly touched onto the slide with a straight down-and-up motion. If the tissue is moved back and forth while on the slide, many of the cells may lyse. If the imprint surface is firm (fibrous), a scalpel can be used to make score marks across the surface after blotting. Once the surface is scored, the imprint is made as described above.

Fine Needle Aspirates

Fine needle aspirates are most commonly used to evaluate mass lesions in the skin, subcutaneous tissue, and tissue within the thorax and abdomen. The primary challenge is obtaining a cellular sample with intact cells. There are several methods for aspiration. Figure 15.3 illustrates two methods for obtaining a fine needle aspirate sample from a cutaneous lesion.

Once the sample is obtained, the next step is to make the slide preparations. Figure 15.4 illustrates several methods for making a cytological preparation.

Once the preparations are made, the slides should be air-dried. There is no reason

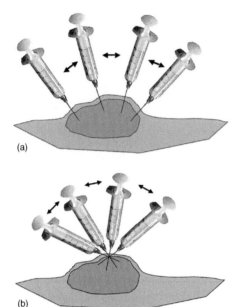

(a)

(b)

Figure 15.3. **(a)** Fine needle aspirate technique using multiple stabs into the mass lesion at separate sites. **(b)** Fine needle aspirate technique using a single entry through skin with redirection of the needle without removing it completely from the mass.

to "fix" cytological preparations. The sample can be stored at room temperature until stained. Do not place the slides in a refrigerator; moisture condensation on the slide will cause lysis of the cells. If the slides are to be submitted to a reference laboratory, the preparations can be sent unstained. It is appropriate to stain a representative slide to insure that there is sufficient cellularity before the sample is sent to the laboratory. The prestained slides should be sent along with the unstained slides because cytological preparations can vary significantly in diagnostic quality.

Cytological preparations should not be transported in the same packaging as formalin-fixed tissue. If the formalin leaks, it will alter the staining quality of the cells and make cytological evaluation of the preparation difficult.

If the fine needle aspirate has a significant amount of blood contamination, as is often the case with liver and spleen aspirates, it is helpful to have a concurrent CBC to help in the interpretation of the number of leukocytes present. If a CBC is not available, a blood film can be used as a comparison. If the sample is to be sent to a reference laboratory, this information can be very helpful to the cytopathologist.

Body Cavity Fluids

Aspiration of body cavity fluids (pleural fluid, peritoneal fluid, pericardial fluid, and joint fluid) is performed to assess the cause of the fluid accumulation. Body cavity fluids should always be collected into an EDTA tube if a full fluid analysis is needed. A complete fluid analysis consists of the following:

- A nucleated cell count
- Protein determination by refractometer
- Cytological evaluation of the fluid

Regardless of how acellular the fluid appears, it should be placed in an EDTA tube to prevent the formation of a fibrin clot that would entrap cells and invalidate the fluid nucleated cell count. If the sample appears cellular (cloudy) and there is concern for sepsis, an additional portion of fluid can be submitted in a sterile container for culture if needed. The apparent cellularity of the fluid predicts the type of slide preparation used for the sample. The blood film method or pull preparation can be used with hemodiluted samples. For highly cellular samples, the pull preparation is most useful. If the sample is only slightly cloudy, a modification of the blood film method can be used. In this method, the push slide is abruptly lifted off the slide before the feathered edge is formed. This method carries the nucleated cells to the edge formed when the push slide is lifted.

(a) Blood Film Preparation

(b) Pull Preparation

(c) Squash Preparation

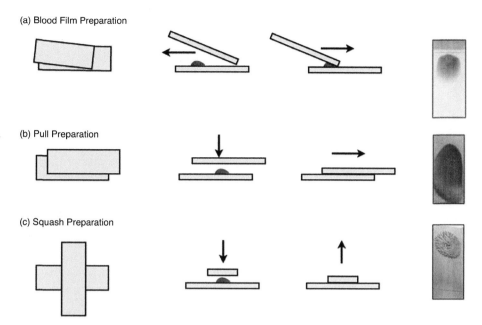

Figure 15.4. Three slide preparation techniques for cytological samples.

In addition, when the sample is clear or just slightly hazy, a portion of the fluid can be centrifuged and a pull preparation can be made from the sediment. This procedure is done after the cell count is performed. If the sediment preparations are submitted to a reference laboratory, they should be clearly labeled. It is helpful to the cytopathologist if a direct preparation of the uncentrifuged fluid is submitted with the sediment preparation as a comparison.

When body cavity fluids are submitted to a laboratory, it is recommended that freshly prepared unstained slides be submitted with the fluid, especially if the sample is sent by an overnight carrier. Cellular detail can deteriorate rapidly over time and any bacteria present, whether a contaminant or a true pathogen, will increase significantly.

Cell counts of fluid samples can be performed using the Unopette™ just as for blood samples. In-house hematology units should not be used to count body cavity fluids because of the increased possibility that the fluid will clog the tubing in the instrument. Thick preparations can be diluted 1:2 to facilitate accurate sampling using the Unopette™ pipette.

Joint fluid is a special case because of the viscosity and contents of the fluid. Normal joint fluid is highly viscous and, in most cases, only a small amount of fluid can be obtained. As with any sample collected into a vacutainer, the vacutainer must be filled at least to 1/4 the volume or the cell count and total protein can be affected by volume dilution and the high specific gravity of EDTA, respectively. If an adequate volume cannot be obtained, a slide preparation and a total protein should be completed and a WBC count performed by directly filling the Unopette™ pipette from the aspiration syringe. It is important to remember that joint fluid contains a large amount of **hyaluronic acid (hyaluronan)** that will precipitate if the Unopette™ dilutent fluid contains acetic

Table 15.2.   Criteria for classifying body cavity fluids.

Type of Fluid	Total Cell Count	Total Protein	Associated Diseases
Transudate	Less than 1000/μl	Less than 2.5 g/dL	Protein-losing renal disease, protein-losing GI disease
Modified transudate	1000–5000/μl	2.5–3.5 g/dL	Cardiac disease, chronic liver disease
Exudate	Greater than 5,000/μl	Greater than 3.5 g/dL	Peritonitis, pleuritis

acid. The mucin clot test, a method for testing joint fluid viscosity, is based on this principle. The Unopette™ system for counting both platelets and leukocytes contains 1% ammonium oxalate and will not cause the joint fluid to precipitate.

Body cavity fluids are categorized by their cellularity and protein level as **transudates**, **modified transudates**, and **exudates**. The criteria for separation of fluids into these categories and the common causes for each type of fluid are given in Table 15.2. Exudate fluid can be further characterized by the cell types present as **suppurative (neutrophils)**, **eosinophilic**, **mixed**, **lymphocytic (chylous)**, **pyogranulomatous**, or **neoplastic**.

Cytology Stains

Romanowsky stains are the standard cytological stains because of their ability to differentially stain the cytoplasm of leukocytes and tissue cells. The most commonly used Romanowsky stains are the modified Wright-Giemsa stains and a fast stain preparation that is alcohol based (Diff-Quik™). All Romanowsky stains contain an acid dye (eosin) and a basic dye (methylene blue, Azure A, or Azure B). The spectrum of colors that are evident with Romanowsky stains is due to the interaction of the acid and basic dyes giving a full range of reds, blues, and purples to specific nuclear and cytoplasmic structures. Cellular

structures that are basic in nature will bind with the acid stain and those that are acid in nature will bind with the basic stains. An example of this is the eosinophil granule. These granules contain a large amount of major basic protein and stain brightly red with the eosin stain. Nuclear material, on the other hand, is highly acidic and stains intensely blue with the basic dyes.

Diff-Quik™ is the most common stain used for in-house cytological examination. When used properly, Diff-Quik™ stain is suitable for most cytological preparations. However, the contents of mast cell granules can leach out resulting in loss of their usual deep basophilic staining properties. This occasionally results in difficulty in identification of mast cell tumors (Figure 15.5).

Modified Wright-Giemsa stains are available that are as quick as the fast stains; they often produce more consistent staining because the staining procedure is based on a set time. Regardless of which type of stain is used, a standard procedure should be followed to produce high-quality slides for evaluation. Stains will deteriorate over time, especially if they are not kept in a closed container to avoid evaporation. In most cases, the intensity of basophilic staining will decrease first or the stain solution will start to precipitate, resulting in a large amount of granular debris on the slide. The stains should be discarded, the staining jars should be cleaned, and fresh stain should be prepared as soon as the quality of the staining begins to decrease. In larger

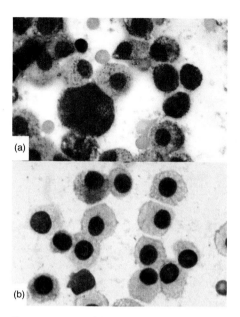

Figure 15.5. Two slide preparations from the same aspirate sample. **(a)** Wrights-Giemsa stain. **(b)** Diff-Quik™ stain: Note the lack of granules in the majority of the mast cells.

laboratories, stains are changed on a routine schedule to reduce the need to restain slides.

Evaluation of Cytological Specimens

When a lesion is examined using cytology, the primary question is whether the lesion is inflammatory or neoplastic. If the lesion is inflammatory, the next question is what type of inflammation is present and is there an infectious agent present. A quality sample with large numbers of intact cells is required to answer each of these questions. Although veterinary technicians are not expected to be cytologists, a background in the type of processes that can be identified by cytology is useful. Technicians should be able to screen cytological preparations for

quality and to recognize inflammatory cells and a variety of infectious agents. A well-trained technician can assist in optimizing the amount of time the veterinarian spends reviewing cytological preparations.

Inflammatory Lesions

Inflammatory lesions are classified based on the cells present in the inflammatory response. The common inflammatory processes are suppurative, granulomatous, pyogranulomatous, and eosinophilic. This classification is based on the predominant cell type in the cytological preparation. Figure 15.6 contains photomicrographs of the different types of inflammatory processes.

The criteria for determination of the type and the common causes for each type of inflammation are presented in Table 15.3. In addition to evaluating the cells present, the background staining characteristics can provide helpful information. High-protein fluids often have a fine to coarsely granular cytoplasm with curved "folds" or protein crescents. Distinct clear vacuoles can be an indicator of lipid in the fluid or aspirate. Cytological preparations from an inflammatory lesion often contain noninflammatory cells such as fibrocytes and cells that line the body cavity from which a fluid sample is taken (mesothelial cells from the thorax and abdomen, synovial cells from joints).

The morphology of the neutrophils in an inflammatory lesion can increase or decrease the suspicion of sepsis. Neutrophils in septic lesions show degenerative changes in their nucleus and are appropriately called degenerative neutrophils. The nuclear changes are loss of nuclear integrity, swelling, and smudging of the nuclear chromatin. Inflammatory lesions with degenerative neutrophils should be closely evaluated for infectious agents. Figure 15.7 illustrates several common infectious agents seen in

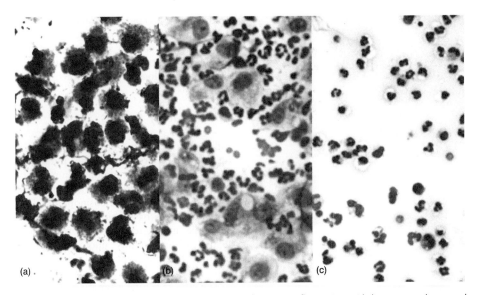

Figure 15.6. **(a)** Eosinophilic inflammation. **(b)** Pyogranulomatous inflammation with large macrophages and neutrophils. **(c)** Neutrophilic inflammation.

cytological preparations. The lack of degenerative neutrophils does not rule out sepsis.

Lesions with large numbers of nondegenerate neutrophils often have tissue necrosis. Samples from a hemorrhagic lesion such as a hematoma can have macrophages that have engulfed erythrocytes (**erythrophagia**) and nucleated cells (**leukophagia**). With chronic hemorrhagic lesions, the macrophages will contain a dark purple staining hemoglobin breakdown product, **hemosiderin**. Figure 15.8 shows several noninflammatory cell types commonly found in cytological preparations.

Neoplastic Lesions

Oncologic cytology is the evaluation of suspected neoplastic lesions. This area of cytology is often the most challenging. When a lesion is determined to be noninflammatory (lacking inflammatory cells) or when atypical tissue origin cells are seen in a preparation that is primarily inflammatory, the cytologist has to determine whether the findings are normal for the site aspirated due to hyperplasia or consistent with neoplasia (benign or malignant). Just as with inflammatory lesions, neoplastic lesions are

Table 15.3. Classifications of inflammatory processes.

Neutrophilic (Suppurative)	Greater than 85% Neutrophils
Eosinophilic	Greater than 50% eosinophils
Granulomatous	Greater than 85% macrophages
Pyogranulomatous	Less than 50% macrophages, greater than 50% neutrophils
Lymphocytic	Greater than 85% lymphocytes

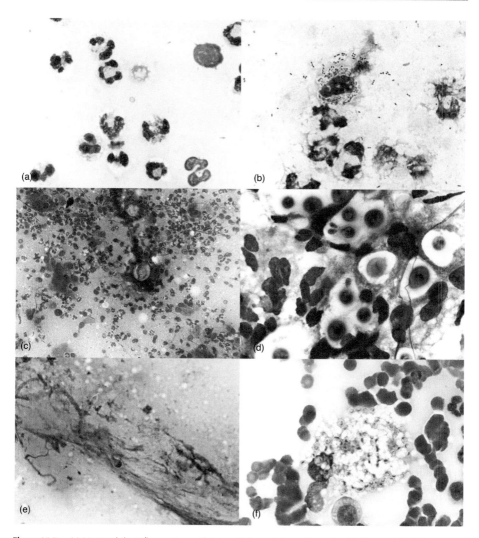

Figure 15.7. **(a)** Neutrophilic inflammation with intracellular rod-shaped bacteria. **(b)** Neutrophilic inflammation with intracellular and extracellular coccoid bacteria. **(c)** Pyogranulomatous inflammation with large *Coccidioides* sp. spherules. **(d)** Neutrophilic inflammation with *Cryptococcus neoformans* yeast. Note the clear halo (capsule) around the yeast bodies and the small oval buds off of two of the yeast bodies. **(e)** Fungal mycelia in a corneal scraping. **(f)** Large macrophage containing small *Histoplasma capsulatum* yeast forms.

classified based on the morphology of the cells present.

Tumors that arise from the supportive tissues of the body are called **mesenchymal tumors**. When it is determined that they

are malignant, they are called sarcomas. If they are considered benign, they are named according to their tissue origin. As an example, a fibroma is a benign proliferation of fibrous connective tissue and a

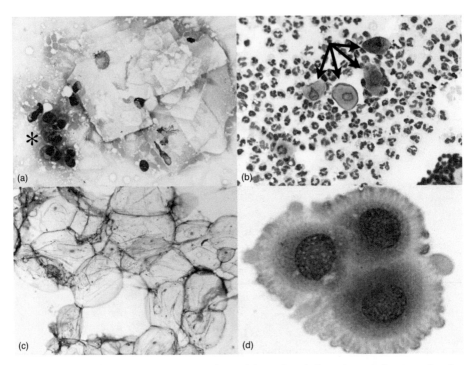

Figure 15.8. **(a)** Small cluster of plasma cells and several large, clear cholesterol crystals (large, angular, clear platelike structures). **(b)** Aspirate of a skin pustule with numerous neutrophils and several squamous epithelial cells. **(c)** A large cluster of large fat cells (adipocytes). **(d)** Three mesothelial cells from the thoracic cavity.

fibrosarcoma is the malignant counterpart to the fibroma.

Tumors that arise from the skin, mucus membranes or glands of the body are epithelial tumors. A **papilloma** is a benign tumor that arises from the squamous epithelial cells of the skin; **squamous cell carcinoma** is a malignant tumor of the squamous cells of the skin. Glandular tumors, such as those that arise in the mammary gland are termed **adenoma** if benign, and **adenocarcinoma** if malignant.

Round cell tumors are the third category of neoplasia. These tumors are mesenchymal in origin but instead of arising from supportive tissues, their origin is individual cells that are found in the interstitial tissues of the body or, in the case of lymphoma, in lymph nodes. Lymphoma, mast cell tumor,

histiocytoma, transmissible venereal tumor, plasma cell tumor, and some melanocytic tumors are considered round cell tumors. Table 15.4 lists several tumors with tissue of origin and benign and malignant forms.

Table 15.4. Tumor terminology.

Tissue of Origin	Benign Form	Malignant Form
Connective tissue	Fibroma	Fibrosarcoma
Bone	Osteoma	Osteosarcoma
Squamous epithelium	Papilloma	Squamous cell carcinoma
Glands	Adenoma	Adenocarcinoma

Table 15.5. Cellular characteristic of tumor types.

Tumor Type	Tendency to Form Clusters	Cell Shape	Cellularity of Sample
Mesenchymal tumors	Low to moderate	Elongate, spindle, oval	Low to moderate
Epithelial tumors	Moderate to high	Polygonal	Moderate to high
Round cell tumors	Low, usually are individual cells	Round to polygonal	High

The criteria that define each of the three categories of neoplasia are general cell shape, cellularity of sample, tendency of the cells to form clusters, the pattern of cell in the clusters, and whether the cells have distinct cytoplasmic borders. Table 15.5 lists the cellular characteristic of mesenchymal, epithelial, and round cell tumors.

The most challenging aspect of oncologic cytology is the differentiation between benign and malignant lesions. Although there are distinct cellular characteristics that assist in this determination, other facts can be just as important as the morphology of the cells. **If the cytological preparation is going to be sent to a laboratory for evaluation, a complete description of the lesion, including specific location and size, is needed.** The location provided should be as specific as possible. For instance, a "skin" mass may be in the skin (cutaneous) or beneath the skin (subcutaneous). An abdominal mass can be on the abdomen, in the abdominal wall, or in the abdominal cavity. Terms such as intraabdominal and intrathoracic are much more specific than simply using the terms *abdominal* and *thoracic* to describe the location of a mass.

The signalment of the animal is also important in helping the cytopathologist develop a differential diagnosis if the cytology is not diagnostic for a specific process. An excellent example of how this information can be crucial for evaluation of a cytological specimen is differentiating a histiocytoma, a benign neoplasm of macrophage origin seen in young dogs, from cutaneous lymphoma, a highly malignant neoplasm of lymphocytes. The morphology of the cells from these two neoplastic processes can be quite similar. If the specimen comes from a 1-year-old dog with a single lesion, the cytopathologist will likely provide a diagnosis of histiocytoma. If the lesion is from an older dog with multiple skin masses, all of which reveal the same cells, the cytopathologist will likely provide a list of potential diagnoses that includes cutaneous lymphoma, with the recommendation that biopsies from multiple masses be submitted for histological evaluation, and possible special stains to help make a final diagnosis.

The cell characteristics that are indications of malignancy are primarily found in the nucleus. Nuclear molding, marked variation in nuclear size (**anisokaryosis**), multiple variably sized nucleoli or large angular nucleoli, and abnormal mitotic figures are findings that indicate a high probability of malignancy. There are few cytoplasmic characteristics that are indicative of malignancy. Increased cytoplasmic basophilia and formation of a large central vacuole that pushes the nucleus to the edge of the cell (signet ring forms) are two cytoplasmic characteristics that are associated with malignant cells. Figure 15.9 shows several photomicrographs of the four types of neoplasia and illustrates several of the cell characteristics that indicate malignancy.

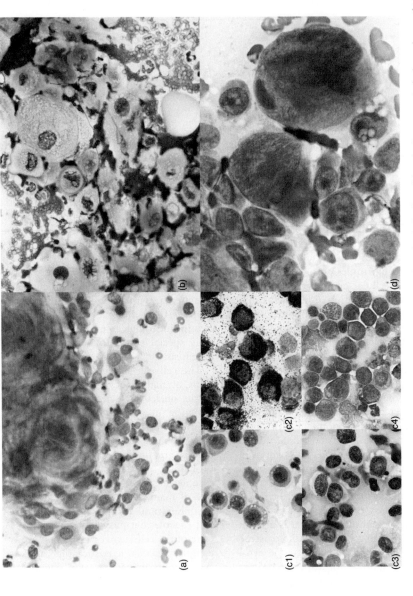

Figure 15.9. **(a)** Soft tissue sarcoma. Note the ill-defined wispy, light blue cytoplasm of the individual cells and the whorling pattern in the large clusters. **(b)** Squamous cell carcinoma. Note the well-defined border and round shape of the neoplastic epithelial cells and the light turquoise color of cytoplasm (keratinized cytoplasm). **(c)** Four types of round cell tumors: (1) transmissible venereal tumor; (2) mast cell tumor; (3) histiocytoma; (4) lymphoma. **(d)** Markedly pleomorphic malignant neoplasm with macronuclei, large abnormal nucleoli, anisocytosis, anisokaryosis.

Although these cellular changes are strongly suggestive of malignancy, it is important to remember that in certain types of malignant lesions, the cells will have none of these characteristics. Apocrine adenocarcinoma of the anal sac is an excellent example of this principle. The epithelial cells that make up this neoplasm are usually very uniform and may have minimal numbers of mitotic figures and no nuclear or cytoplasmic changes suggestive of the highly aggressive nature of these lesions.

On the other hand, hyperplasia, the process of increased cell production in response to inflammation, is associated with changes in the hyperplastic cells that mimic neoplasia. When inflammation is present in a lesion, extreme care must be taken to prevent overinterpretation of changes in the tissue cells present. Fibrocytes in chronic inflammatory lesions can show several characteristics of malignancy, especially in young animals. Mesothelial cells, the cells that line the body cavities, often proliferate and can form variable-sized clusters with significant anisokaryosis when fluid is present in these cavities. Even the most experienced cytopathologist may not be able to differentiate hyperplasia from neoplasia in some cases.

Appendix A

Tables

Table A.1. Normal values for canine and feline complete blood count.

Test	Canine Normal Range	Feline Normal Range
Packed cell volume	35–55%	24–44 %
Hemoglobin	12–18 g/dL	8–15 g/dL
Mean corpuscular volume (MCV)	60–77 fL	39–55 fL
Mean corpuscular hemoglobin concentration	32–36 g/dL	30–36 g/dL
White blood cell count	6,000–17,000 n/μL	5,500–19,500 n/μL
Neutrophils, seg	3,000–11,400 n/μL	2,500–12,500 n/μL
Neutrophils, bands	0–300 n/μL	0–300 n/μL
Lymphocytes	1,000–4,000 n/μL	1,500–7,000 n/μL
Monocytes	150–1350 n/μL	0–850 n/μL
Eosinophils	100–750 n/μL	0–750 n/μL
Platelets	220,000–550,000 n/μL	300,000–500,000 n/μL

Table A.2.   Normal values for canine/feline chemistry.

Test	Canine Normal Range	Feline Normal Range
Alkaline phosphatase	10–150 U/L	0– 62 U/L
Albumin	3.1–4.5 g/dL	2.4–4.1 g/dL
ALT (SGPT)	5–60 U/L	27–76 U/L
Amylase	500–1500 IU/L	500–1500 IU/L
AST (SGOT)	5–55 U/L	5–55 U/L
GGT	0–14 U/L	0–6 U/L
Albumin	2.5–3.6 g/dL	2.3–3.3 g/L
Total protein	5.1–7.8 g/dL	5.9–8.5 g/L
Globulin	2.8–4.5 g/dL	3.6–5.6 g/L
Total bilirubin	0–0.4 mg/dL	0–0.4 mg/dL
BUN	7–27 mg/dL	15–34 mg/dL
Creatinine	0.4–1.8 mg/dL	0.8–2.3 mg/dL
Glucose	60–125 mg/dL	70–150 mg/dL
Calcium	8.2–12.4 mg/dL	8.2–11.8 mg/dL
Phosphorus	2.1–6.3 mg/dL	3.0–7.0 mg/dL
Chloride (Cl)	105–115 mEq/L	111–125 mEq/L
Sodium (Na)	141–156 mEq/L	147–156 mEq/L
Potassium (K)	4.0–5.6 mEq/L	3.9–5.3 mEq/L

Table A.3.   Normal blood gas levels.

Test	Canine Normal Range	Feline Normal Range
Blood pH	7.35–7.45	7.35–7.45
pCO2	34–40 mm HG	34–40 mm HG
Anion gap	15–25 mEq/L	15–25 mEq/L
Base excess	0 – +6	−5 – +2
Sodium bicarbonate	20–24 mg/dL	16–20 mg/dL

Table A.4.   Normal clotting times.

Test	Canine Normal Range	Feline Normal Range
Prothrombin times (PT)	12–17 sec	15–23 sec
Partial prothrombin times (aPTT)	71–102 sec	70–120 sec

Table A.5. Emergency diagnostics.

Clinical Test	Normal
Packed cell volume	Canine >55% Feline >45 % Canine <35 % Feline <25 %
Serum	Straw-colored
Buffy coat	Buffy coat should be <1 % but visible
Total protein	Canine: 5–7.2 g dL Feline: 5.8–8.5 g/dL
Albumin	Canine: 3.1–4.5 g dL Feline: 2.4–4.1 g/dL
Blood glucose	Canine: 60–115 mg/dL Feline: 60–130 mg/dL
Electrolytes	Sodium (Na)—Canine: 142–150 mEq/L Feline: 147–162 mEq/L
	Chloride (Cl) —Canine: 105–117 mEq/L Feline: 114–126 mEq/L
	Potassium (K)—Canine: 4.5–5.4 mEq/L Feline: 3.7–5.2 mEq/L
Lactate	Lactate >3 (Normal can vary from machine to machine.)
Clotting times	PT Canine: 71–102 sec Feline 70–120 sec
	aPTT Canine: 12–17 sec Feline: 15–23 sec
Blood pressure	Systolic = 100–140 mm Hg

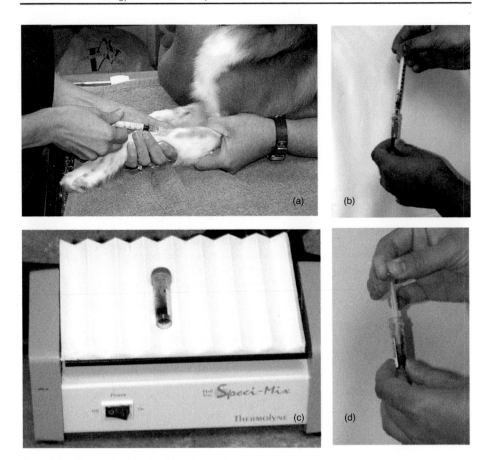

Figure A.1.   How to draw blood and handle samples.

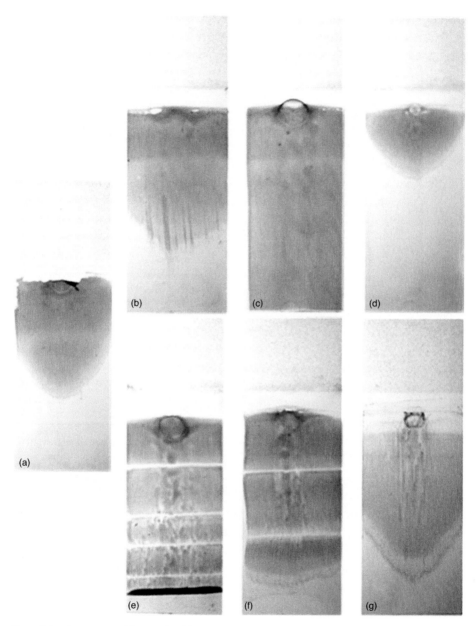

Figure A.2. Components of the complete blood count.

Table A.6. Common poikilocytosis and associated diseases.

Type of Cell Noted	Shape of Cell	Disease
Echinocytes (crenated cell)	Numerous uniformly distributed tent-shaped spikes	Artifact of drying, snake bite, dehydration, inherited erythrocyte defects
Acanthocytes	Irregularly spaced thin spikes with knoblike tips; no central pallor	Prominent numbers: liver disease, renal disease, hemangiosarcoma Small numbers: iron deficiency, microangiopathy
Eccentrocytes	Dense eccentric displacement of hemoglobin with a clear edge	Oxidative injury, onion toxicity
Schistocytes	Small irregular fragments of the erythrocyte	Microangiopathy, iron deficiency, hemangiosarcoma, valvular stenosis
Spherocytes	Small dense cells with no central pallor	Large numbers: hemolytic anemia Small numbers: microangiopathy, iron deficiency.
Keratocytes	Surface blisters that rupture to form small horn-lick extensions.	Iron deficiency, microangiopathy, liver disease
Burr cells (ovalo-echinocytes)	Elongate cells with spikes similar to a crenated cell	Feline liver disease, renal disease.

Table A.7. Causes of regenerative and nonregenerative anemia.

Regenerative Anemia	Nonregenerative anemia
Blood loss (trauma, coagulation defects) Immune-mediated hemolytic anemia Oxidative hemolytic anemia Erythroparasites	Bone marrow neoplasia (leukemia, nonmarrow [metastatic]) Bone marrow fibrosis Infectious disease (FeLV, chronic ehrlichiosis) Toxicity Chronic renal disease (lack of erythropoietin)

Table A.8. Semiquantitation method for polychromasia.

Degree of Polychromasia	Number of Polychromatophilic Cells/1000×
Few	0–1
1+	1–2 (dog), 0–1 (cat)
2+	2–3 (dog), 1–2 (cat)
3+	3–6 (dog), 2–4 (cat)
4+	6 (dog), >4 (cat)

Table A.9. Reticulocyte percentages and absolute numbers and corresponding degree of regeneration.

Reticulocyte Percentage (Corrected)	Absolute Reticulocyte	Degree of Regeneration
<1% (dog), <0.4% (cat)	<60,000 (Dog), <40,000 (cat)	No regeneration
1–4% (dog), 0.5–2% (cat)	60–150,000 (dog), 40–70,000 (cat)	Mild regeneration
5–20% (dog), 3–4% (cat)	150–300,000 (dog), 70–100,000(cat)	Moderate regeneration
<20% (dog), >4% (cat)	300,000 (dog), >100,000 (cat)	Marked regeneration

Table A.10. Diseases associated with erythrocyte destruction and mechanisms.

Immune-mediated hemolytic anemia	Extravascular hemolysis: macrophage removal of antibody coated erythrocytes	Intravascular hemolysis: lysis of erythrocytes by antibody on the cell surface
Heinz body anemia/eccentrocyte-associated anemia	Oxidative injury to hemoglobin (zinc, drugs); extravascular hemolysis: macrophage removal of erythrocytes with Heinz bodies	
Erythroparasites	Extravascular hemolysis: macrophage removal of infected erythrocytes (antibodies to the organism contributes to the phagocytosis)	Intravascular hemolysis: lysis of heavily infected Erythrocytes (may be antibody mediated)
Hypophosphatemia	Extravascular hemolysis: removal of erythrocytes with oxidative injury	Intravascular hemolysis, possibly due to disruption of erythrocyte metabolism.

Table A.11. Hereditary diseases associated with hemolytic anemia.

Disease	Common Breed
Hereditary spherocytosis	Miniature schnauzers, Alaskan malamutes
Pyruvate kinase deficiency	Basenji, beagles, West Highland white terriers, cairn terriers, miniature poodles
Phosphofructokinase deficiency	English springer spaniels, American cocker spaniel

Table A.12. Types of polycythemia.

Relative	Dehydration, splenic contraction
Absolute primary	Polycythemia vera
Absolute secondary	Hypoxia (general)
	Renal hypoxia (renal masses)
	Erythropoietin-like substance produced by nonrenal neoplasia

Table A.13. Clinical diagnostics that help to monitor kidney function.

Element	Element That Suggests Decreased Glomerular Filtration	Other Factors That Elevate Element Level	Factors Indicating That True Renal Azotemia Is Occurring
BUN	Azotemia BUN >26 mg/dL (Canine) BUN >34 mg/dL (Canine)	GI bleeding High protein meal	USG >1.015
Creatinine	Azotemia Crea >1.3 mg/dL (Canine) Crea >2.2 mg/dL (Feline)	None	USG >1.015
Phosphorus	P >5.5 mg/dL (Canine) P >7.0 mg/dL (Feline)	Disease that affects calcium and phosphorus balance.	Increased phosphorus must be in association with elevated BUN/creatinine and low USG.
Potassium	K <4.0 mEq/L (Canine) K <3.7 mEq/L (Feline)	Any disease that can cause fluid loses (i.e., vomiting, anorexia, or diarrhea may lower body potassium)	Decreased potassium must be in association with elevated BUN/creatinine and low USG.
Potassium	K >5.4 mEq/L (Canine) K >5.2 mEq/L (Feline)	Hypoadrenocorticism (Addison's Dz)	Increased potassium must be in association with acute elevations of BUN/creatinine and urinary obstruction. CAN BE ACUTELY LIFE THREATENING
Albumin	Alb <3.1 g/dL (Canine) Alb <2.4 g/dL (Feline)	Liver disease Bleeding Gastrointestinal Dz	Possible early warning of impending renal disease. Low albumin must be associated with a true renal proteinuria (see Ch 11).

Table A.14. Risks of patients with reduced hepatic function.

Liver Function	Concern of Dysfunction
Detoxification	*Hepatic encephalopathy*: Development of neurologic symptoms secondary to improper detoxification of microbes and toxins, which remain in the body affecting the central nervous system.
	Physical symptoms due to build of toxins and bilirubin: Increased toxins can produce nausea, anorexia, depression, vomiting, diarrhea, weakness, and weight loss.
Formation of building blocks	*Anemia*: Lack of red blood cell precursors
	Increased clotting time: The liver produces clotting factors that finalize clot formation.
	Hypoalbuminemia: Due to lack of blood albumin, the body can shift fluid from the vascular supply to the tissue, increasing fluid accumulation in the body producing ascites, edema, and pulmonary edema (with patients on IV fluids).
Glucose storage	*Hypoglycemia* (rare)

Table A.15.   Algorithm: Diagnosis of renal disease.

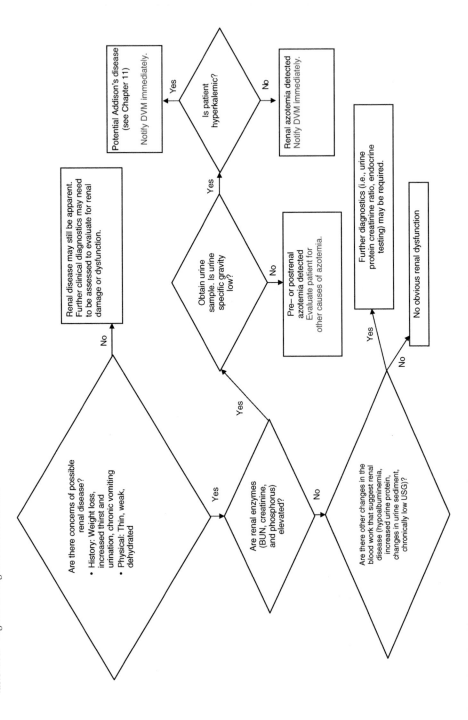

Table A.16. Algorithm for hepatic clinical diagnostics.

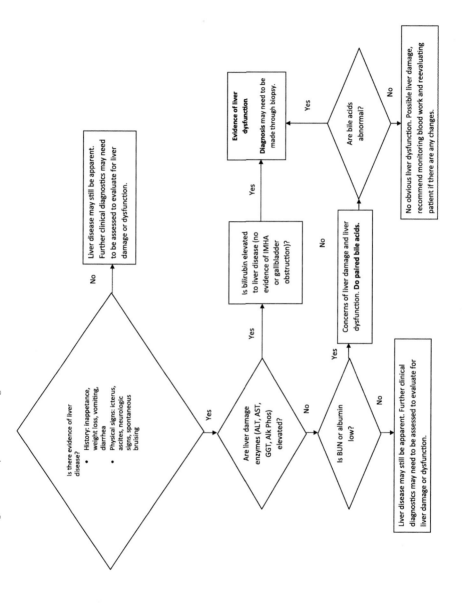

Table A.17. Algorithm for clinical diagnostics of the gastrointestinal system.

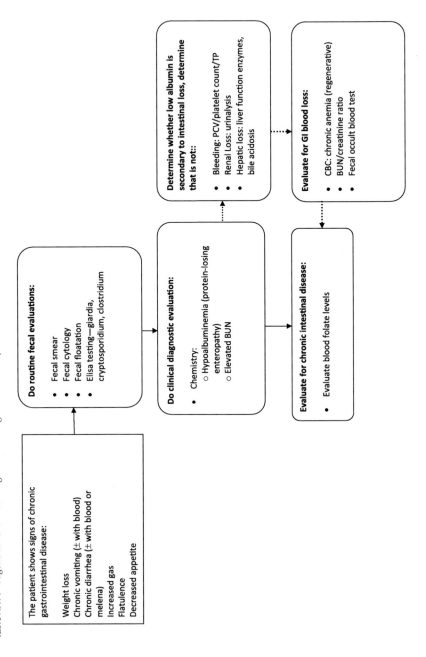

The patient shows signs of chronic gastrointestinal disease:

Weight loss
Chronic vomiting (± with blood)
Chronic diarrhea (± with blood or melena)
Increased gas
Flatulence
Decreased appetite

Do routine fecal evaluations:

- Fecal smear
- Fecal cytology
- Fecal floatation
- Elisa testing—giardia, cryptosporidium, clostridium

Do clinical diagnostic evaluation:

- Chemistry:
  o Hypoalbuminemia (protein-losing enteropathy)
  o Elevated BUN

Determine whether low albumin is secondary to intestinal loss, determine that is not::

- Bleeding: PCV/platelet count/TP
- Renal Loss: urinalysis
- Hepatic loss: liver function enzymes, bile acidosis

Evaluate for chronic intestinal disease:

- Evaluate blood folate levels

Evaluate for GI blood loss:

- CBC: chronic anemia (regenerative)
- BUN/creatinine ratio
- Fecal occult blood test

Table A.18. Algorithm for acute exocrine pancreatic patient (pancreatitis)—canine

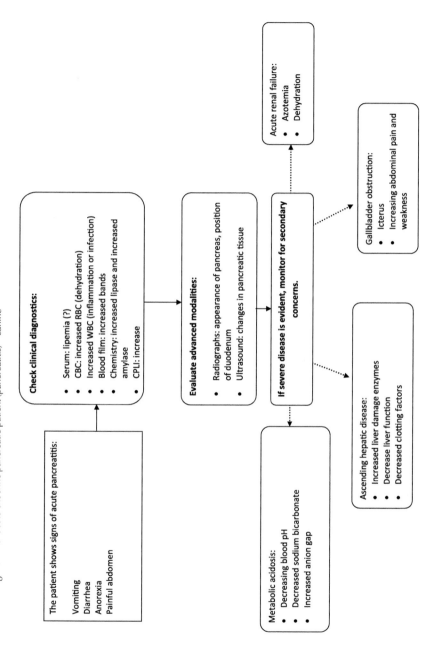

The patient shows signs of acute pancreatitis:

Vomiting
Diarrhea
Anorexia
Painful abdomen

Check clinical diagnostics:

- Serum: lipemia (?)
- CBC: increased RBC (dehydration)
- Increased WBC (inflammation or infection)
- Blood film: increased bands
- Chemistry: increased lipase and increased amylase
- CPLI: increase

Evaluate advanced modalities:

- Radiographs: appearance of pancreas, position of duodenum
- Ultrasound: changes in pancreatic tissue

If severe disease is evident, monitor for secondary concerns.

Acute renal failure:
- Azotemia
- Dehydration

Gallbladder obstruction:
- Icterus
- Increasing abdominal pain and weakness

Ascending hepatic disease:
- Increased liver damage enzymes
- Decrease liver function
- Decreased clotting factors

Metabolic acidosis:
- Decreasing blood pH
- Decreased sodium bicarbonate
- Increased anion gap

Table A.19. Algorithm for chronic exocrine pancreatic patient (pancreatitis)—canine.

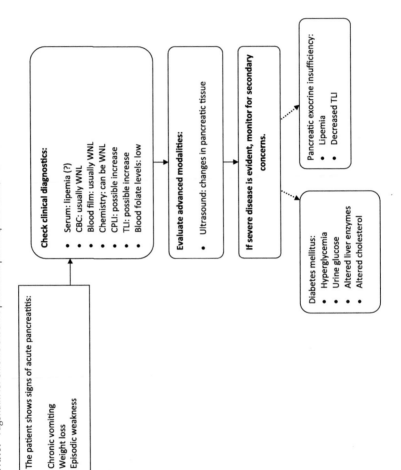

The patient shows signs of acute pancreatitis:

Chronic vomiting
Weight loss
Episodic weakness

Check clinical diagnostics:

- Serum: lipemia (?)
- CBC: usually WNL
- Blood film: usually WNL
- Chemistry: can be WNL
- CPLI: possible increase
- TLI: possible increase
- Blood folate levels: low

Evaluate advanced modalities:

- Ultrasound: changes in pancreatic tissue

If severe disease is evident, monitor for secondary concerns.

Diabetes mellitus:

- Hyperglycemia
- Urine glucose
- Altered liver enzymes
- Altered cholesterol

Pancreatic exocrine insufficiency:

- Lipemia
- Decreased TLI

Table A.20.   Algorithm for acute/chronic exocrine pancreatic patient (pancreatitis)—feline.

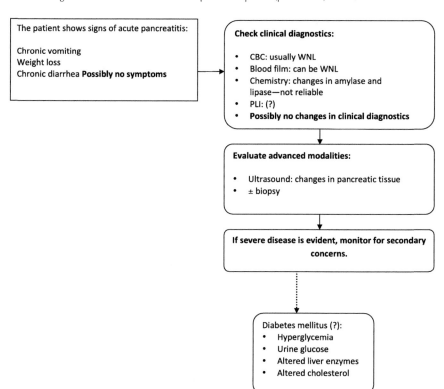

The patient shows signs of acute pancreatitis:

Chronic vomiting
Weight loss
Chronic diarrhea **Possibly no symptoms**

Check clinical diagnostics:

- CBC: usually WNL
- Blood film: can be WNL
- Chemistry: changes in amylase and lipase—not reliable
- PLI: (?)
- **Possibly no changes in clinical diagnostics**

Evaluate advanced modalities:

- Ultrasound: changes in pancreatic tissue
- ± biopsy

If severe disease is evident, monitor for secondary concerns.

Diabetes mellitus (?):
- Hyperglycemia
- Urine glucose
- Altered liver enzymes
- Altered cholesterol

Table A.21. Algorithm for endocrine pancreatic patient (Diabetes mellitus).

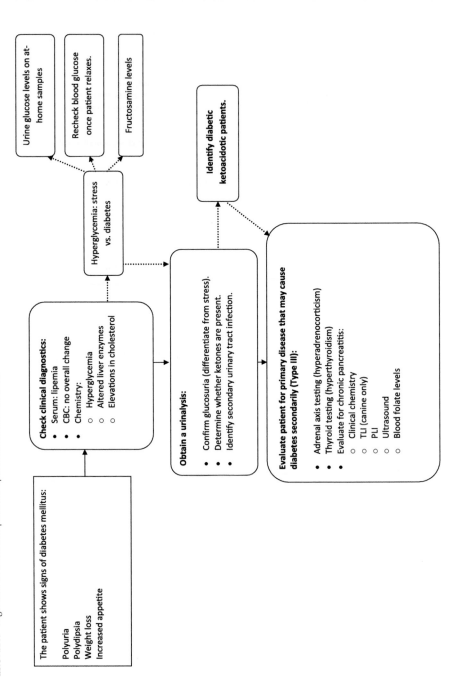

Table A.22. Electrolyte abnormalities, their causes and secondary concerns.

Element	Normal Finding	Presence of Abnormality Suggests
Sodium	Canine: 142–150 mEq/L Feline: 147–162 mEq/L	**Hyponatremia:** Associated with loss of solute from vomiting and diarrhea and hypoadrenocorticism. **Evaluate potassium levels.** **Hypernatremia:** Associated with increased intake and loss of large quantities of fluids.
Potassium	Canine : 4.0–5.4 mEq/L Feline: 3.7–5.2 mEq/L	**Hypokalemia:** Associated with chronic gastrointestinal loss (vomiting/diarrhea), chronic renal disease, and long-term IV fluid therapy. Severe hypokalemia can be associated with treatment of the DKA patient. **Hyperkalemia:** • **Artifactual hyperkalemia** can be associated with specific breeds (Japanese canine breeds), chronic intestinal/parasitic disease, and severe abnormalities in white blood cell count and platelet count. • **Disease:** Associated with hypoadrenocorticism and urinary obstruction. **Evaluate sodium level.**
Chloride	Canine : 105–117 mEq/L Feline: 114–126 mEq/L	**Hypochloremia:** Closely associated with causes of hyponatremia and loss of solute. **Hyperchloremia:** Closely associated with hypernatremia and increased intake and loss of large quantities of fluids.
Calcium	Canine : 9.2–11.2 mg/dL Feline: 7.2–11.4 mg/dL	**Hypocalcemia:** Associated with eclampsia, acute/chronic renal failure, and ethylene glycol intoxication. **Hypercalcemia:** Associated with specific types of cancers, acute renal failure, overproduction of parathyroid hormone, hypoadrenocorticism, specific rodenticides, and specific types of infection.
Phosphorus	Canine : 2.3–5.5 mg/dL Feline: 3.0–7.0 mg/dL	**Hypophosphotemia:** Associated with the treatment of the DKA patient. If levels <1.0 mg/dL, hypophosphotemia can produce a hemolytic anemia. **Hyperphosphotemia:** Associated with decreased excretion of phosphorus from the kidneys secondary to renal disease and failure. Can be also associated with diseases that produce severe prerenal and postrenal azotemia (see Chapter 5).

Table A.23. Elements of the urine and their meanings.

Urinary Element	Normal Finding	Presence of Abnormality Suggests
Urine specific gravity	Canine >1.025 Feline >1.035	Decreased urine specific gravity can suggest the kidneys' inability to concentrate urine. This can occur simply due to increased fluid intake (oral, IV fluids) or be secondary to renal or hormonal diseases.
Urine glucose (glucosuria)	Negative	**Artifact:** Decreased USG <1.005 can hide glucosuria on the reagent strip (false negative). Further contamination of the urine may produce a false positive. **Disease:** True glucosuria can suggest diabetes mellitus or in some cases stressed patients with hyperglycemia and glucosuria (see Chapter 7).
Urine ketones (ketonuria)	Negative	**Artifact:** Test checks for only one kind of ketone, so a negative does not always rule out ketonuria. Further, false positive ketone reactions can be seen with administration of captopril, D-penicillamine, iopronin, and cystine. **Disease:** A true ketonuria is always present with glucosuria and suggests the patient is suffering from diabetes ketoacidosis (see Chapter 7).
Conjugated bilirubin (bilirubinuria)	Negative	**Artifact:** Can show false positive based on contamination of sample. **Disease:** Can support evidence of liver disease, IMHA, or gallbladder obstruction in the patient.
Blood (hematuria)	Negative	**Artifact:** Test can show positive for blood, hemoglobin, or myoglobin. Disease that affect red blood cell destruction (e.g., IMHA) or muscle disease can cause increased release of hemoglobin or myoglobin and make this test falsely positive. To help confirm the diagnosis of hematuria, the urine supernatant should be evaluated after the urine is spun. Patients with true hematauria will have a clear supernatant because the cells have been condensed into the pellet. **Disease:** Hematuria suggests disease that produces bleeding into the urinary bladder—e.g., urinary tract infections, urinary crystals and stones (urolithiasis), or bladder/renal tumors.
Protein (proteinuria)	Canine: negative to trace Feline: negative	**Artifact:** Artifactual proteinuria can occur if urine pH is alkaline (>7.5). **Disease:** The presence of urine protein (especially in diluter urine) can suggest evidence of urinary tract disease or renal disease with glomerular damage.
Sediment— white blood cells	(<0–2 WBC hpf)	Evidence of increased white blood cells supports the presence of infection or inflammation within the urinary tract. Increased white blood cells are most commonly observed with urinary tract infections.
Sediment— red blood cells	(<0–3 WBC hpf)	Evidence of increased red blood cells supports the presence of bleeding within the bladder suggesting urinary tract infections, chronic bladder crystals or stones, or bladder or renal tumors.

Table A.23. (*Continued*)

Urinary Element	Normal Finding	Presence of Abnormality Suggests
Sediment—epithelial cells	(<1–2/lpf)	Increased evidence of epithelial cells can suggest the presence of some types of bladder cancer. When noted, the urinary sample should be sent to the lab for cytological evaluation.
Sediment—bacteria or fungus	None	True bacterial or fungal elements in the urine supports renal or urinary tract infection. If these elements are noted, the type of microorganism should be documented. Further, the presence of white blood helps to further confirm that an infection is evident.
Casts—hyaline	Negative	Caused by Protenuria
Casts—granular	Negative	The presence of granular casts can suggest renal tubular necrosis.
Casts—cellular	Negative	**Uncommon.** Their presence does suggest serious renal disease and its cause is dependent on the type of cell found. Red blood cell casts suggest renal hemorrhage or inflammation, whereas white blood cell casts suggest renal infection.
Casts— waxy	Negative	If evident, they can suggest chronic renal tubular damage secondary to chronic kidney disease.
Casts— fatty	Negative	Can suggest patients with increased fat content, most notably in the cat.
Crystals—triple phosphate	Negative	**Artifact:** Can precipitate out in samples that sit for too long at room temperature. **Disease:** Suggestive of crystallization of magnesium, phosphorus, and ammonia out of dietary elements in urine with an alkaline pH.
Crystals—calcium oxalate	Negative	**Artifact:** Can precipitate out in samples that sit for too long at room temperature. **Disease:** Suggestive of crystallization of calcium and oxalate out of dietary elements in urine with an acidic pH.
Crystals—monohydrate calcium oxalate	Negative	These crystals are evident with ethylene glycol intoxication (antifreeze) within the first 8 hours of ingestion.
Crystals—bilirubin	Negative	Normal findings in concentrated urine in canines. Can suggest diseases that produce hyperbilirubinemia (e.g., liver disease, gallbladder obstruction, or IMHA).
Crystals—ammonium biurate crystals	Negative	Evident in patients with liver dysfunction and in dalmatians.

Table A.24. Flowchart A—Evaluating urine color, turbidity, and specific gravity.

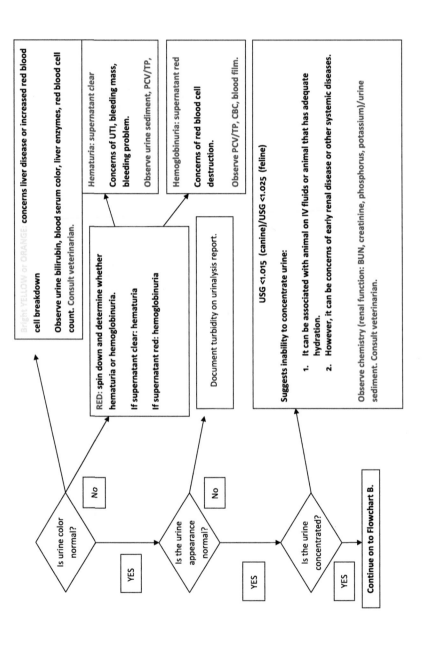

Is urine color normal?

No →

Bright YELLOW or ORANGE: concerns liver disease or increased red blood cell breakdown

Observe urine bilirubin, blood serum color, liver enzymes, red blood cell count. Consult veterinarian.

RED: spin down and determine whether hematuria or hemoglobinuria.

If supernatant clear: hematuria

If supernatant red: hemoglobinuria

Hematuria: supernatant clear

Concerns of UTI, bleeding mass, bleeding problem.

Observe urine sediment, PCV/TP,

Hemoglobinuria: supernatant red

Concerns of red blood cell destruction.

Observe PCV/TP, CBC, blood film.

YES

Is the urine appearance normal?

No →

Document turbidity on urinalysis report.

YES

Is the urine concentrated?

No →

USG <1.015 (canine)/USG <1.025 (feline)

Suggests inability to concentrate urine:

1. It can be associated with animal on IV fluids or animal that has adequate hydration.
2. However, it can be concerns of early renal disease or other systemic diseases.

Observe chemistry (renal function: BUN, creatinine, phosphorus, potassium)/urine sediment. Consult veterinarian.

YES

Continue on to Flowchart B.

Table A.24. *(Continued)*

Flowchart B—Evaluating urine chemistry—key factors.

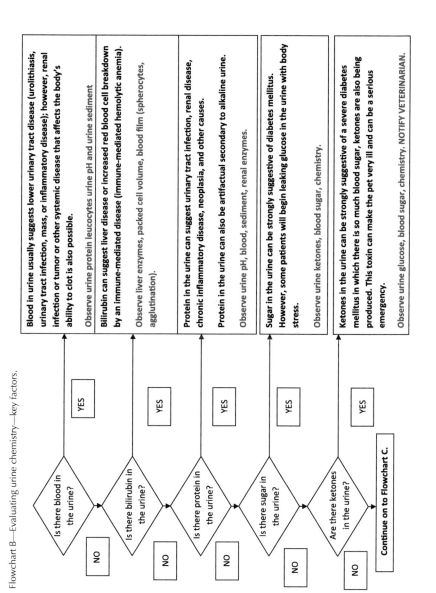

Is there blood in the urine? — YES → **Blood in urine usually suggests lower urinary tract disease (urolithiasis, urinary tract infection, mass, or inflammatory disease); however, renal infection or tumor or other systemic disease that affects the body's ability to clot is also possible.**

Observe urine protein leucocytes urine pH and urine sediment

Is there bilirubin in the urine? — YES → **Bilirubin can suggest liver disease or increased red blood cell breakdown by an immune-mediated disease (immune-mediated hemolytic anemia).**

Observe liver enzymes, packed cell volume, blood film (spherocytes, agglutination).

Is there protein in the urine? — YES → **Protein in the urine can suggest urinary tract infection, renal disease, chronic inflammatory disease, neoplasia, and other causes.**

Protein in the urine can also be artifactual secondary to alkaline urine.

Observe urine pH, blood, sediment, renal enzymes.

Is there sugar in the urine? — YES → **Sugar in the urine can be strongly suggestive of diabetes mellitus. However, some patients will begin leaking glucose in the urine with body stress.**

Observe urine ketones, blood sugar, chemistry.

Are there ketones in the urine? — YES → **Ketones in the urine can be strongly suggestive of a severe diabetes mellitus in which there is so much blood sugar, ketones are also being produced. This toxin can make the pet very ill and can be a serious emergency.**

Observe urine glucose, blood sugar, chemistry. NOTIFY VETERINARIAN.

NO (through each)

Continue on to Flowchart C.

Table A.24. *(Continued)*

Flowchart C—Evaluating urine sediment.

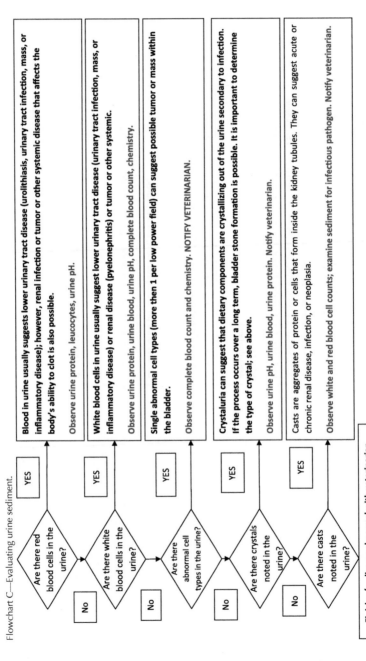

Are there red blood cells in the urine?

YES → **Blood in urine usually suggests lower urinary tract disease (urolithiasis, urinary tract infection, mass, or inflammatory disease); however, renal infection or tumor or other systemic disease that affects the body's ability to clot is also possible.**

Observe urine protein, leucocytes, urine pH.

No ↓

Are there white blood cells in the urine?

YES → **White blood cells in urine usually suggest lower urinary tract disease (urinary tract infection, mass, or inflammatory disease) or renal disease (pyelonephritis) or tumor or other systemic.**

Observe urine protein, urine blood, urine pH, complete blood count, chemistry.

No ↓

Are there abnormal cell types in the urine?

YES → **Single abnormal cell types (more then 1 per low power field) can suggest possible tumor or mass within the bladder.**

Observe complete blood count and chemistry. NOTIFY VETERINARIAN.

No ↓

Are there crystals noted in the urine?

YES → **Crystalluria can suggest that dietary components are crystallizing out of the urine secondary to infection. If the process occurs over a long term, bladder stone formation is possible. It is important to determine the type of crystal; see above.**

Observe urine pH, urine blood, urine protein. Notify veterinarian.

No ↓

Are there casts noted in the urine?

YES → **Casts are aggregates of protein or cells that form inside the kidney tubules. They can suggest acute or chronic renal disease, infection, or neoplasia.**

Observe white and red blood cell counts; examine sediment for infectious pathogen. Notify veterinarian.

No ↓

Finish u/a: discuss abnormal with veterinarian.

Table A.25. Algorithm: Diagnosis of Cushing's disease.

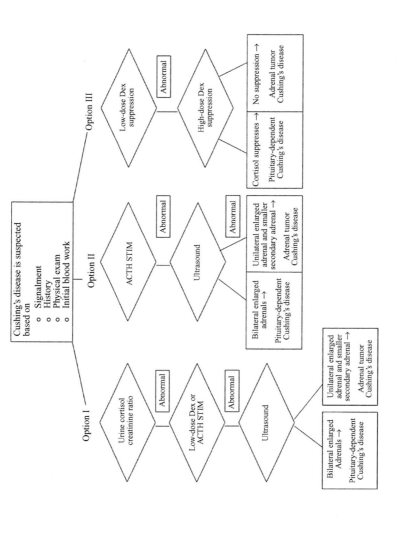

Table A.26. Algorithm: Causes of acidosis.

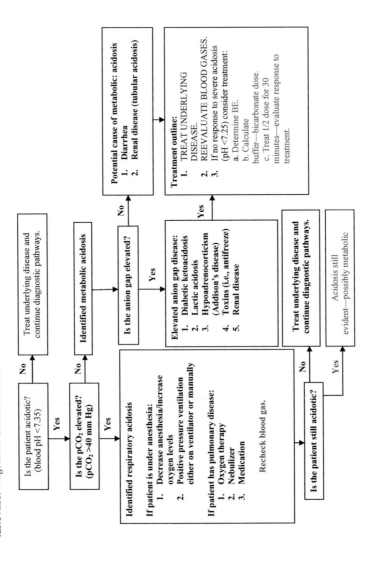

Table A.27. Primary hemostasis.

Test	Outcome
Platelet count	Decreased platelet number will affect the body's ability to produce the initial clot (<40,000/µL).
Platelet function tests	Sent out to lab when presented with a bleeding animal with normal platelet number and normal clotting times.
Buccal mucosal bleeding	Done as an in-house lab test for lack of von Willebrand's factor (von Willebrand's disease)

Table A.28. Secondary hemostasis.

Test	Cascade Affected	Possible Causes
Prolonged PT Normal aPTT	Extrinsic cascade	Factor VII deficiency
Normal PT Prolonged aPTT	Intrinsic cascade	Factor VIII or IX deficiency
Prolonged PT Prolonged aPTT	Both cascades	Multiple factor deficiencies: Vitamin K antagonism (rat poison) Liver disease DIC Inherited Dz: Factor X Thrombin

Table A.29.   Overview of Code I diagnostics.

Clinical Test	Outcome	Other Diagnostics	Cause/Action
Packed cell volume	Canine >55% Feline >45 %	Should be a marked increase in albumin/ total protein.	Dehydration: Notify veterinarian. Prepare patient for aggressive fluid therapy.
	Canine <35 % Feline <25 %	Check purple top for clot or agglutination. Check albumin/total protein for decrease.	Notify veterinarian. Causes: • Blood loss • Chronic anemia of disease • IMHA • Artifact
Serum	Straw-colored	If hemolyzed, check PCV for anemia; check purple top for agglutination. If icteric, check PCV for anemia and purple top for agglutination. Check patient for physical jaundice. If lipemic, check medical history for the last time patient ate.	Document all changes to serum and notify veterinarian.
Buffy coat	Buffy coat should be <1% but visible	Check white blood cell count and blood film.	Decreased buffy coat: viral infection/immunosuppression Increased buffy coat: infection/inflammation/cancer
Total protein	Canine: 5–7.2 g dL Feline: 5.8–8.5 g/dL	Low total protein: Evaluate PCV/TP, albumin. High total protein: Evaluate PCV/TP, albumin, and globulin.	Low total protein can suggest bleeding, renal disease, liver disease, chronic intestinal disease, or possibly disease that produces a decreased immune response (low immunoglobulin). High total protein: dehydration or disease that produces an increased immune response (high immunoglobulin)
Albumin	Canine: 3.1–4.5 g dL Feline: 2.4–4.1 g/dL	Low albumin: Evaluate PCV/TP, clotting times, urinalysis, renal enzymes, liver enzymes. High albumin: Evaluate PCV/TP.	Low total protein can suggest bleeding, renal disease, liver disease, chronic intestinal disease. High total protein: dehydration

Table A.29. *(Continued)*

Clinical Test	Outcome	Other Diagnostics	Cause/Action
Blood glucose	Canine: 60–115 mg/dL Feline: 60–130 mg/dL	Low blood glucose: Check white blood cell count/blood film. Increased blood glucose: urinalysis, fructosamine, chemistry.	Low blood sugar: sepsis Notify veterinarian immediately. Increased blood glucose: diabetes mellitus, stress
Electrolytes	Sodium (Na): Canine: 142–150 mEq/L Feline: 147–162 mEq/L Chloride (Cl): Canine: 105–117 mEq/L Feline: 114–126 mEq/L Potassium (K): Canine: 4.5–5.4 mEq/L Feline: 3.7–5.2 mEq/L	Chemistry Urinalysis	Decrease in electrolytes is caused by vomiting, diarrhea, fluid therapy. Increase in potassium: FLUTD, hypoadrenocorticism Notify veterinarian immediately.
Lactate	Lactate >3 (Although normal can vary from machine to machine.)	Blood gas	Increased lactate supports decreased ability to oxygenate tissue (perfusion). This makes the tissue burn energy through fermentation and lactate builds up. Serial lactates serve as a monitor of how the body is responding to treatment to increased oxygenation of blood and body perfusion.
Clotting times	PT: Canine: 71–102 sec Feline 70–120 sec aPTT: Canine: 12–17 sec Feline: 15–23 sec	Increased clotting times: Evaluate PCV/TP, albumin, CBC (platelet count).	Increased clotting times support the patient's ability to clot blood (see Chapter 13). Notify veterinarian immediately.
Blood pressure	Systolic >100–140 mm Hg		Any abnormalities, notify veterinarian immediately.

Table A..30. Algorithm: Evaluating blood film on emergency patients.

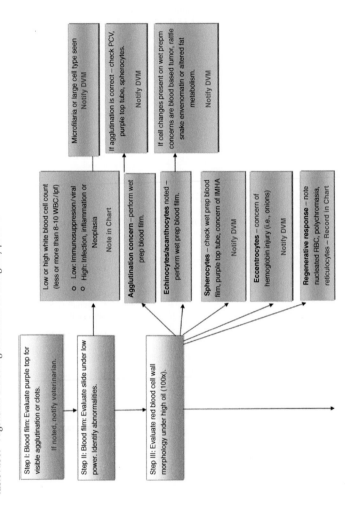

Step I: Blood film: Evaluate purple top for visible agglutination or clots.

If noted, notify veterinarian.

Step II: Blood film: Evaluate slide under low power. Identify abnormalities.

Step III: Evaluate red blood cell wall morphology under high oil (100x).

Low or high white blood cell count (less or more than 8-10 WBC/lpf)

o Low: Immunosuppresion/viral
o High: Infection, inflammation or Neoplasia

Note in Chart

Agglutination concern – perform wet prep blood film.

Echinocytes/acanthocytes noted – perform wet prep blood film.

Spherocytes – check wet prep blood film, purple top tube, concern of IMHA

Notify DVM

Eccentrocytes – concern of hemoglobin injury (i.e, onions)

Notify DVM

Regenerative response – note nucleated RBC, polychromasia, reticulocytes – Record in Chart

Microfilaria or large cell type seen
Notify DVM

If agglutination is correct – check PCV, purple top tube, spherocytes.

Notify DVM

If cell changes present on wet prepm concerns are blood based tumor, rattle snake envenomatin or altered fat metabolism.

Notify DVM

Table A.30. *(Continued)*

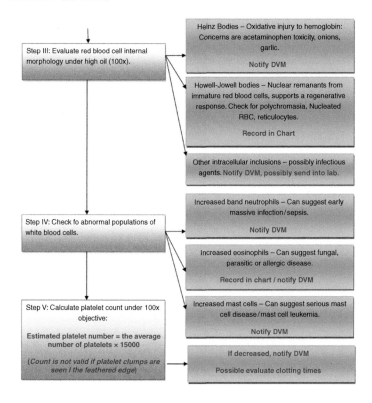

Table A.31. Complications associated with fine needle aspiration.

Complication	Site
Pneumothorax	Lung
Hemorrhage	Liver, kidney, spleen, lung
Tumor seeding	Neoplastic lesions
Bacteremia	Abscess (internal or external)
Sepsis	Abscess (internal or external)

Table A.32. Criteria for classifying body cavity fluids.

Type of Fluid	Total Cell Count	Total Protein	Associated Diseases
Transudate	Less than 1000/μL	Less than 2.5 g/dL	Protein-losing renal disease, protein-losing GI disease
Modified transudate	1000–5000/μL	2.5–3.5 g/dL	Cardiac disease, chronic liver disease
Exudate	Greater than 5000/μL	Greater than 3.5 g/dL	Peritonitis, pleuritis

Table A.33. Classifications of inflammatory processes.

Neutrophilic (suppurative)	Greater than 85% neutrophils
Eosinophilic	Greater than 50% eosinophils
Granulomatous	Greater than 85% macrophages
Pyogranulomatous	Less than 50% macrophages, greater than 50% neutrophils
Lymphocytic	Greater than 85% lymphocytes

Table A.34. Tumor terminology.

Tissue of Origin	Benign Form	Malignant Form
Connective tissue	Fibroma	Fibrosarcoma
Bone	Osteoma	Osteosarcoma
Squamous epithelium	Papilloma	Squamous cell carcinoma
Glands	Adenoma	Adenocarcinoma

Table A.35. Cellular characteristic of tumor types.

Tumor Type	Tendency to Form Clusters	Cell Shape	Cellularity of Sample
Mesenchymal tumors	Low to moderate	Elongate, spindle, oval	Low to moderate
Epithelial tumors	Moderate to high	Polygonal	Moderate, to high
Round cell tumors	Low, usually are individual cells	Round to polygonal	High

Appendix B

Clinical Pathology for the Veterinary Team DVD Instructions

Introduction: The following material is to help each participant get the full enjoyment of the interactive case studies which expose the student to medical history, physical examination findings, clinical diagnostics and virtual slides to help them create problem lists for each case. It is important to understand that the goal of the program is to have the student practice their knowledge in an interactive environment; it is the responsibility of the veterinarian to interpret medical history and physical exam findings, recommend clinical diagnostics and evaluate the outcome.

Computer Requirements: The Power-Point program can work on any PC/ Mac computer with a CD-ROM / DVD drive. In order to utilize the virtual slide portion of this program, Mac Users will need to have software that allows the computer to emulate a PC Desktop environment. Scan scope should then be loaded onto this portion of the MAC interface and be utilized with the DVD.

Opening the Program:

Step I: Open Program Button and Click on my computer

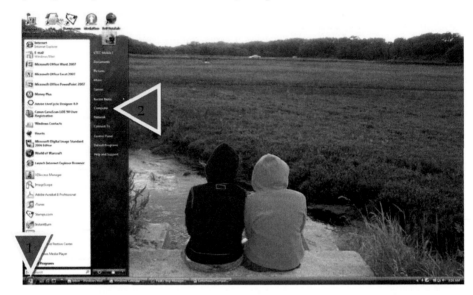

Step II: Click on DVD / CD-ROM Drive and open DVD:

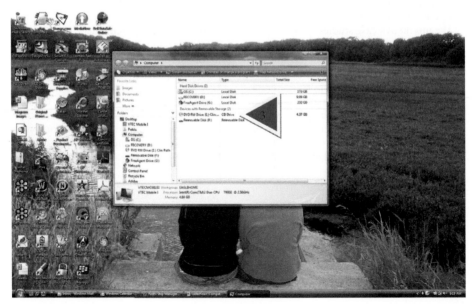

Step III: Open (Double Click) *"Clin Path CD Folder"*

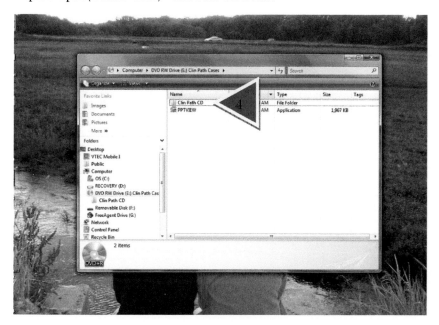

Step IV: Double Click on PPTVIEW File

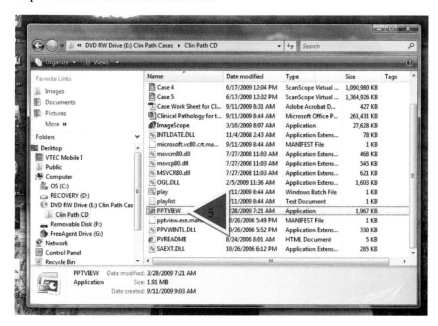

Step V: Select Clinical Pathology for the Vet Team CD-ROM – It will begin the show.

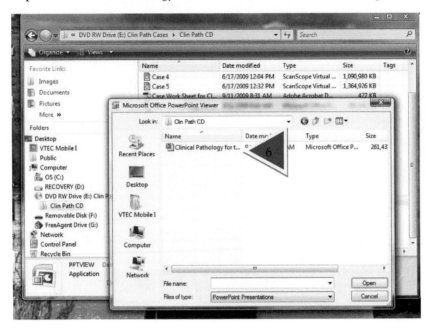

Instructions on how to load Scan Scope unto your computer to view Virtual Slides

Step I: Select Install Scan Scope Tab on Program.

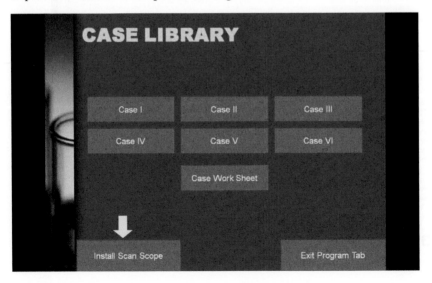

Most computers will have a pop-up which asks do you want to open this file, please click on "ok".

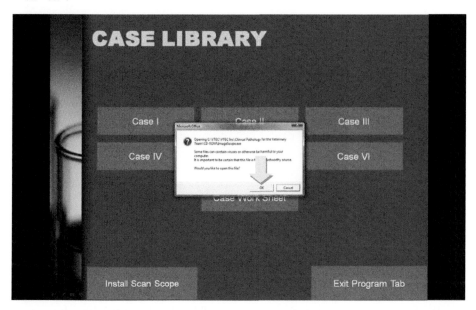

Step II: Program will open, select next.

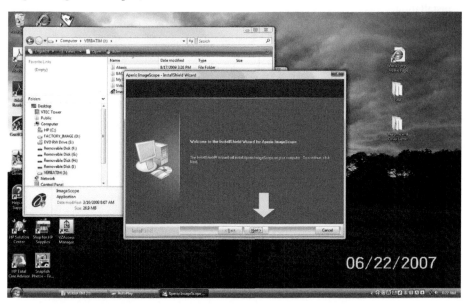

Step III: Read Aperio software agreement, accept agreement and select next.

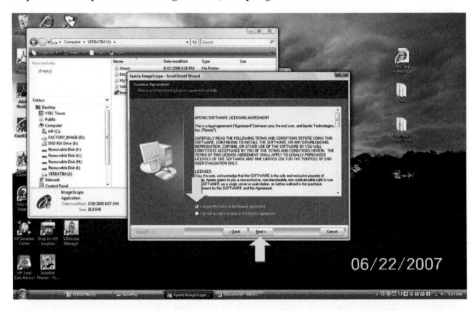

Step IV: Aperio will make suggestion where file will be placed on hard drive. It is a very small file and in most cases it will place the file on the hard drive. Selecting next will start installation.

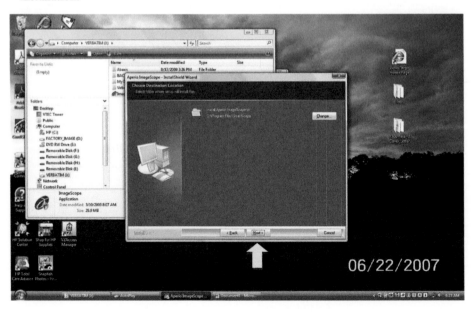

Step V: Finish - When done, exit out of scan scope and re-select the CD-ROM program

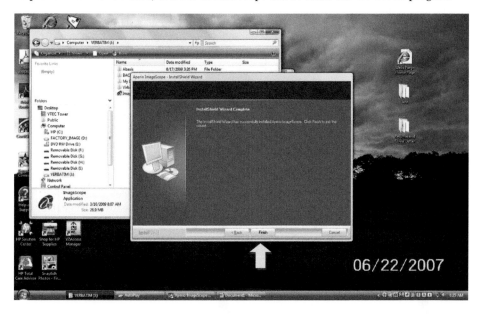

Step VI: Reselect CD-ROM Tab and enter program

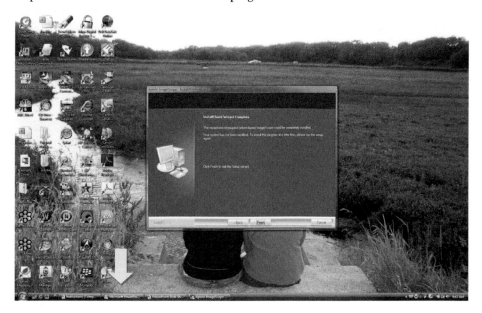

To Navigate in the PowerPoint Environment: Once in the PowerPoint environment, you will be able to navigate through each slide by clicking on selected tabs to move forward, answer a question, evaluate a heart rhythm, or make choices where to go in the program. To fully enjoy this process, please follow the following guidelines to navigate in this environment:

1. **When the program begins, you may get a Macro Warning:** These programs contain commands called "Macros" that allow the participant to move throughout the environment, listen to sound files and view image files contained on these CDs. These are not meant to affect your computer or its ability to function. In order to use the CD-ROMS you will need to select to activate the macros in this presentation.

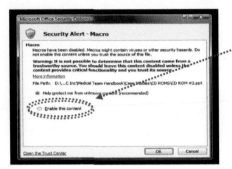

In order to view this program properly, please select enable Macro and click okay. The program will then load and run normally.

2. **When selecting a tab, make sure that the mouse arrow has change to a small hand before left clicking the mouse button.** This will select the proper tab, and will not move you one slide forward in the program.

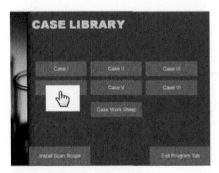

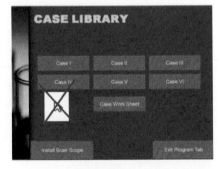

CORRECT WAY – The mouse has gone from arrow to hand, showing you are selecting the proper tab.

Incorrect Way: In this image the arrow has not changed into the hand and by clicking the mouse will move the program forward one slide only.

3. When using the mouse, you inadvertently click or use the dial to move one slide forward. If you do inadvertently move to the next slide and are out of place, simply right click the mouse which will bring up the following options:

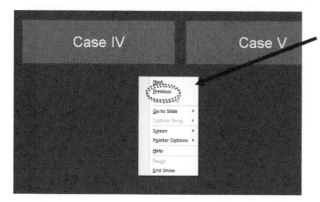

By right clicking the mouse, the following options become available, please highlight "Previous" and click with the left mouse button. This will move you back one slide space.

4. There is no narration for the slide: On occasion the PowerPoint may not initiate the narrative sequence; to restart the narration process, simply click the left mouse button once.

Appendix C

Case Worksheet for Clinical Pathology Cases

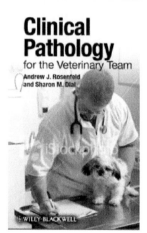

Clinical Pathology
for the Veterinary Team
Andrew J. Rosenfeld
and Sharon M. Dial

WILEY-BLACKWELL

Andrew J Rosenfeld, DVM and Sharon Dial, DVM

Case #_____

Signalment: _____

Chief Complaint: _____

Triage Exam:
- Temperature:
- Pulse:
- Respiration:
- Capillary Refill Time:
- Mucus Membrane Color:
- Hydration:
- Mentation:

Where should the patient be placed?

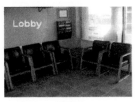 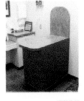 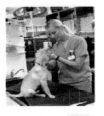 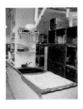

Lobby   **Exam**   **Tech**   **Emergency**

History Questions:

1.
2.
3.
4.
5.
6.
7.
8.
9.
10.

Full Exam – List Abnormal

Cardiovascular	
Respiratory	
Abdomen	
Lymph Nodes	
Integument (skin)	
Eyes / Ears / Nose / Throat	
Reproductive System	
Musculoskeletal System	
Neurologic System	

Problem List – Based on History & Physical Examination

1.
2.
3.
4.
5.
6.
7.
8.
9.
10.

Which Testing Protocols are indicated?

☐ Level I Diagnostic:
    1. PCV / TP
    2. Blood Film
    3. Blood Glucose
    4. BUN
    5. Blood Gas
    6. Electrolytes
    7. Clotting Time

Full Diagnostic:
    ☐ CBC
    ☐ Chemistry
    ☐ Urinalysis
    ☐ Electrolytes
    ☐ Clotting Times
    ☐ Blood Gas
    ☐ ACTH Response Test
    ☐ Thyroid Screen
    ☐ Other:_____

PCV / TP / Serum

Clinical Test	Finding	Concern

Complete Blood Count: If not getting a complete blood count with this case, please move to the next table.

Clinical Test	Finding	Concern

Blood Film:

Concern	Observation
Agglutination vs. Rouleaux	
Red Blood Cell Membrane	
Red Blood Cell Internal Architecture	
Abnormal Red Blood Cells	
Impression of White Blood Cell Population	
Platelet Evaluation	

Chemistry: If not getting a complete chemistry with this case, please enter the emergency data base associated with chemistry.

Clinical Test	Finding	Concern
BUN		
Glucose		

Electrolytes:

Clinical Test	Finding	Concern

Urinalysis: If not getting a urinalysis with this case, please move to the next table.

Clinical Test	Finding	Concern

Blood Gas: If not getting a blood gas with this case, please move to the next table.

Clinical Test	Finding	Concern

Clotting Time: If not getting a clotting time with this case, please move to the next table.

Clinical Test	Finding	Concern

Problem List – Based on Clinical Diagnostic Testing

    1.
    2.
    3.
    4.
    5.
    6.
    7.
    8.
    9.
   10.

Other Testing – Please write down other tests that should be evaluated:

    1.
    2.
    3.
    4.
    5.
    6.
    7.
    8.
    9.
   10.

   Comments:

Additional Resources

Although there are many excellent technical books to help create a good medical library, the authors suggest the following.

Books

The 5 Minute Veterinary Consult: Canine and Feline, Third Edition. Tilley, L., and Smith, F. Wiley-Blackwell, Ames, IA, hardcover, 2009. ISBN #978-0-7817-7063-7.

Essentials of Veterinary Hematology. Jain, Nemi C. Wiley-Blackwell, Ames, IA, 1st edition, 1993. ISBN #978-0812114379.

Clinical Anatomy and Physiology for Veterinary Technicians. Colville, T., and Bassert, J. Mosby, St. Louis, 2002. ISBN #0-323-00819-4.

Veterinary Hematology: Atlas of Common Domestic and Non-Domestic Species. Reagan, William J.; Irizarry Rovira, Armando R.; and DeNicola, Dennis B. Wiley-Blackwell, Ames, IA, 2d edition, 2008. ISBN #978-0813828091.

Veterinary Hematology and Clinical Chemistry: Text and Clinical Case Presentations Set. Thrall, Mary Anna; Baker, Dale C.; Campbell, Terry W.; and DeNicola, Dennis B. Lippincott Williams & Wilkins, St. Louis, 1st edition, 2004. ISBN #978-0781768504.

The Veterinary Medical Team Handbook. Rosenfeld, A. Wiley-Blackwell, Ames, IA, 2007. ISBN #978-0-7817-5759-1.

Online Resource

Virbac University: Online programs in dentistry, dermatology, endocrine, heartworm, and management: www.virbacuniversity.com

Glossary

Acanthocytes (Chapter 4): A change in the red blood cell population noted by irregular, spiky projections of the red blood cell membrane that have variable-sized knobs on the spike tips and generally do not retain an area of central pallor.

Acidosis (Chapter 12): A condition that occurs when the patient's blood pH is <7.35.

ACTH (adrenocorticotrophic hormone) (Chapter 11): A hormone produced by the pituitary gland that stimulates the adrenal gland to produce cortisol.

Activated partial thromboplastin time (aPTT) (Chapter 13): An assay that evaluates the intrinsic clotting pathway.

Addisonian crisis (Chapter 11): A life-threatening crisis produced by a lack of aldosterone in the body.

Adenocarcinoma (Chapter 15): A malignant tumor that arises from glandular tissue.

Adenoma (Chapter 15): A benign tumor that arises from glandular tissue.

Adrenal cortex (Chapter 11): The outer tissue layer responsible for producing different types of steroids for maintenance of blood glucose, electrolytes, and sex hormone production.

Adrenal medulla (Chapter 11): The tissue in the middle of the gland that is responsible for producing epinephrine and norepinephrine to assist the central nervous system in times of crisis (fight or flight response).

Alanine aminotransferase (ALT) (Chapter 6):: An enzyme is responsible for the conversion of 2-oxoglutarate to pyruvate and glutamate in the liver cells (hepatocytes).

Albumin (Chapter 5): Protein produced in the liver and released in the bloodstream to carry molecules throughout the body.

Albuminuria (Chapter 5): The presence of albumin in the urine.

Aldosterone (Chapter 8): The hormone responsible for the reabsorption of sodium and expulsion of potassium in the distal convoluted tubules in the kidney.

Alkaline phosphatase (SALP or ALP) (Chapter 6):: A phosphatase present within the liver, intestine, bone, kidneys, and placenta. On most chemistry panels, alkaline phosphatase activity represents the combined activity of all combined tissue alkaline phosphatase levels.

Amylase (Chapter 7): A pancreatic enzyme that cleaves large sugar molecules into smaller single sugars.

Amyloidosis (Chapter 6): An accumulation of an inert protein in the liver that can chronically destroy normal liver tissue.

Anemia (Chapter 2): Decreased circulating erythrocytes.

Anemia of chronic disease (Chapter 14): Severe anemia produced by a chronic disease that decreases the body's ability to regenerate red blood cells.

Angiotension (Chapter 5): A hormone in the body that is activated by renin to help cause a potent constriction of the blood vessels.

Anion (Chapter 12): A negatively charged ion.

Anion gap (AG) (Chapter 12): The unmeasured anions in a serum sample.

Anisokaryosis (Chapter 15): A marked variation in nuclear size.

Aplastic anemia (Chapter 4): A severe anemia produced by a lack of progenitor cells within the bone marrow.

Ascites (Chapter 6): An accumulation of fluid in the abdomen secondary to liver dysfunction.

Aspartate aminotransferase (AST) (Chapter 6):: An intracellular enzyme, present in all cells, which has higher levels of activity in muscle and liver cell damage.

Azotemia (Chapter 5): Increased blood ammonia.

Babesiosis (Chapter 4): An infection or disease caused by *Babesia canis* or *Babesia gibsoni*, internal erythroparasites within the erythrocyte cytoplasm.

Band neutrophil (Chapter 4): An immature neutrophil whose nucleus is not segmented.

Basophil (Chapter 3): A white blood cell that is rarely seen in peripheral blood. Although its function is unknown, fungal and parasitic infections increase the basophil population.

Basophilic stippling (Chapter 4): Stippling of erythrocytes that is characterized by fine basophilic reticulum seen on Wright-Giemsa stain. The reticulum is aggregated RNA (just as in reticulocytes) and is seen most occasionally seen in regenerative anemia.

Bernard-Soulier syndrome (Chapter 13): A genetic platelet function disorder that inhibits platelets from adhering to von Willebrand's factor.

Bile acids (Chapter 6): Chemicals produced by the liver to help emulsify fat within the small intestine.

Bile canaliculi (Chapter 6): Small channels in the liver that take detoxified toxins into the gallbladder.

Bilirubin (Chapters 5, 6): A toxic metabolite produced from the red blood cell destruction in the spleen and the breakdown of hemoglobin.

Blood folate levels (Chapter 7): A measure of the blood levels of the B vitamin folate. Low levels can help support chronic gastrointestinal disease and bacterial overgrowth.

Blood urea nitrogen (BUN) (Chapter 5): Blood urea nitrogen as an amalgamation of two ammonia molecules produced by the liver.

Bowman's capsule (Chapter 5): A specialized filtering structure within the renal cortex.

Buccal mucosal bleeding time (Chapter 13): A clinical diagnostic commonly done to screen dogs for von Willebrand's disease. A small shallow cut is made in the mucosal surface of the upper lip and the time from the initial cut to cessation of bleeding is recorded.

BUN/creatinine ratio (Chapter 8): A ratio of blood levels of BUN/creatinine, which can help support the concern of gastrointestinal bleeding.

Burr cells (ovalo-echinocytes) (Chapter 4): Oval-shaped cells with numerous small spikes similar to those on crenated cells commonly seen in diseases associated with changes in the erythrocyte membrane lipid. Feline hepatic lipidosis is commonly associated with increased numbers of burr cells.

Calcium (Chapter 8): A body element that is needed by almost every cell in the body to control cellular activity, aid in muscular contraction, help heart function, and aid nerve conduction as well as other body functions.

Carbon dioxide (Chapter 12): A gas produced through respiration and excreted by the body as a toxin.

Casts (urinary) (Chapter 9): Formed elements that are literally casts of the tubules within the renal cortex in which they form.

Cation (Chapter 12): A positively charged ion.

Chediak-Higashi syndrome (Chapter 4): A rare inherited disorder that is characterized by abnormal leukocytes.

Chloride (Chapter 8): An abundant anion in the extracellular fluid.

Cholelithe (Chapter 6): Gallbladder stones.

Chylothorax (Chapter 4): An accumulation of lymphocyte-rich fluid (lymph) in the thoracic cavity.

Chylous (Chapter 15): A milky fluid consisting of lymph and emulsified fat extracted from chyme by the lacteals during digestion and passed to the bloodstream.

Coagulation factors (Chapter 13): Chemicals produced by the liver that function in the formation of fibrin.

Coagulopathy (Chapter 13): The inability of the blood to clot.

Coefficient of variance (Chapter 1): The ratio of the standard deviation of a data set divided by the average of the same data set. A low ratio suggests good precision.

Compensating metabolic alkalosis (Chapter 12): A condition that occurs when a patient suffering from metabolic acidosis increases respiration (lowers pCO_2) to lower blood carbon dioxide levels and try to decrease overall acid levels in the body.

Convoluted tubules (Chapter 5): A structure within the nephron that functions to aggressively reabsorb all of the necessary nutrients back into the bloodstream.

Cortisol (Chapter 11): A steroid hormone produced by the adrenal gland.

Creatinine (Chapter 5): An amino acid that is a metabolite of muscle creatinine, which is produced in the body during normal muscle metabolism.

Crenated erythrocytes (Chapter 4): An artifact seen on blood films when the blood film dries slowly.

Crystaluria (Chapter 5): The presence of crystals in urine.

Cytauxzoon felis (Chapter 4): A protozoan erythroparasite of cats similar in appearance to *Babesia gibsoni*.

D-dimer assays (Chapter 13): A clinical diagnostic to identify increased degradation of fibrin.

Degenerate left-shift (Chapter 3): The release of immature neutrophils from the bone marrow.

Demodex (Chapter 15): A skin mite.

Dermatophytic fungi (Chapter 15): A fungal infection of the skin.

Diabetes mellitus (Chapter 7): A disease produced by decreased insulin production in the body.

Diabetic Ketoacidotic (Chapter 7): A condition of severe diabetes wherein patients produce a toxin called acetone.

Disseminated intravascular coagulopathy (DIC) (Chapter 14): A syndrome seen in association with many disease processes, which places the patient in a procoagulation state.

Dohlé body (Chapter 4): Angular, basophilic cytoplasmic inclusions, also indicating toxic change.

Eccentrocytes (Chapter 4): Erythrocytes with fusion of a portion of the cell membrane that causes the hemoglobin to be pushed to the side.

Echinocytes (Chapter 4): Erythrocytes with spiky protrusions from their surface.

Eclampsia (postparturient hypocalcemia) (Chapter 8):: A serious condition of the dog shortly after pregnancy due to increased demands of blood calcium secondary to lactation.

Elastase (Chapter 3): A neutrophilic enzyme used on foreign debris and bacteria to break down tissue.

Elliptocytosis (Chapter 3): A genetic disease due to a defect in one of the network proteins in which the cells are oval-shaped rather than the normal biconcave disc.

Endothelial cells (Chapter 13): Cells that line all blood vessels.

Eosinophil (Chapter 3): A white blood cell that is involved in response to parasitic infections, fungal disease, some protozoal diseases, allergies, and immune-complex disease.

Eosinophilia (Chapter 4): An increased number of circulating eosinophils in the blood.

Epinephrine (Chapter 11): A neurochemical transmitter involved with the sympathetic nervous system.

Epistaxis (Chapter 12): Bleeding from the nose.

Erythrocyte (Chapter 2): A red blood cell.

Erythrophagia (Chapter 15): Body macrophages that have engulfed erythrocytes.

Erythropoiesis (Chapter 3): Production of red blood cells in the bone marrow.

Erythropoietin (Chapter 3): A hormone produced from the kidneys at a constant rate to maintain the normal rate of erythropoiesis.

Ethylene glycol (Chapter 5): A toxin found in antifreeze that can cause severe renal disease.

Extrinsic pathway (Chapter 13): A stepwise chemical reaction that is involved in the formation of a fibrin clot.

Exudates (Chapter 15): A fluid obtained from a body cavity with a total protein of >3.5 mg/dL and a total cell count of >5000 cell/μL.

Feline lower urinary tract disease (FLUTD) (Chapter 10): A syndrome of urinary tract disease and obstruction in the feline.

Fermentation (Chapter 14): The process of producing energy from glucose in a low oxygen environment.

Fibrin (Chapter 13): The mortar that is formed during secondary hemostasis, which is the process of stabilizing the platelet plug. Fibrin holds the platelets together.

Fibrinogen (Chapter 13): The protein precursor that circulates in the plasma.

Fibrinogen degradation product (FDP) (Chapter 13): A clinical diagnostic to identify increased degradation of fibrin.

Fibrinolysis (Chapter 13): The breakdown of blood clots that is the opposing mechanism that reestablishes blood flow after the vessel is repaired by dissolving the clot that is obstructing the vessel.

Fight or flight response (Chapter 11): A group of behaviors associated with the release of epinephrine from the sympathetic nervous system.

Folate (Chapter 8): A B vitamin produced in the intestine of the canine and feline.

Gallbladder (Chapter 6): A collecting site for deactivated toxins within the liver.

Gamma-glutamyltransferase (GGT) (Chapter 6): An indicator of gallbladder obstruction or lack of bile flow. GGT is an intracellular enzyme responsible for cleaving C-terminal glutamyl groups from one substrate or molecule to another, and it is thought to be involved in pathways used to protect cells from oxidative injury.

Gangliosidosis (Chapter 4): A rare inherited disease that is characterized by abnormal leukocytes.

Glanzmann's thrombasthenia (Chapter 13):: A genetic platelet function disorder that inhibits platelets from adhering to each other.

Glomerular filtration (Chapter 5): The rate at which renal glomeruli filter blood.

Glomeruli (Chapter 5): Specialized structures within the renal cortex that remove toxins from the bloodstream.

Glucagon (Chapter 7): A pancreatic enzyme that responds to lower blood sugar levels to stimulate the conversion of glycogen and fat back into glucose.

Glucose (Chapter 7): Blood sugar.

Glucosuria (Chapter 7): Glucose present in the urine.

Glycogen (Chapter 6): A form of glucose stored by the liver.

Glycolysis (Chapter 3): The metabolic pathway that converts glucose, $C_6H_{12}O_6$, into pyruvate, $C_3H_3O_3$. The free energy released in this process is used to form the high energy compounds, ATP (adenosine triphosphate).

Granulomatous disease (Chapter 11): Several infectious diseases, primarily fungal, whereby normal tissue is replaced by inflammatory cells that form multiple granulomas.

Granulopoiesis (Chapter 3): Production of neutrophils, eosinophils, and basophils in the bone marrow.

Heinz body (Chapter 4): A cellular inclusion that is formed by oxidative injury to the hemoglobin in the erythrocyte and are most common in the cat. The hemoglobin denatures and adheres to the cell membrane forming a spherical light or clear staining inclusion that may extend out from the cell membrane.

Hemangiosarcoma (Chapter 14): A type of tumor arising from blood vessels.

Hematemesis (Chapter 7): Vomiting blood.

Hematocrit (Hct) (Chapter 2): A calculated measurement of the percent of red blood cells present in the blood.

Hematology (Chapter 3): The study of the cellular components of blood.

Hematoma (Chapter 5): A very large collection of blood under the skin, usually caused by traumatic blood draw.

Hematopoiesis (Chapter 3): The production of blood cells.

Hematuria (Chapter 9): Blood present in the urine.

Hemoconcentration (Chapter 9): An increase in the red blood cell population of blood secondary to dehydration.

Hemoglobin (Hgb) (Chapter 2): A chemical compound within the red blood cell that has the ability to carry oxygen and carbon dioxide.

Hemoglobinemia (Chapter 4): A process whereby red blood cells are lysed within the vessels and hemoglobin is released into the bloodstream.

Hemoglobinuria (Chapter 9): The presence of hemoglobin in the urine.

Hemogram (Chapter 2): The collection of specific measurements that allow the veterinarian to evaluate a patient's erythrocytes, leukocytes, and platelets.

Hemolysis (Chapter 5): Lysis of red blood cells, releasing hemoglobin into the serum.

Hemosiderin (Chapter 15): A hemoglobin breakdown product.

Hemostasis (Chapter 13): The process of turning free-flowing blood into a stationary clot.

Hepatic encephalopathy (Chapter 6): A neurologic syndrome caused by the buildup of toxins entering the central nervous system that have not been properly detoxified by the liver.

Hepatic lipidosis (Chapter 6): A disease syndrome that occurs commonly in the cat and horse (pony) when these animals have a disease entity that produces a profound anorexia. The animals shunt large amounts of fat into the liver to transform it into sugar. This fatty infiltration affects the ability of the liver to function.

Hepatitis (Chapter 6):: The activation of the immune system by some foreign antigen within the liver.

Hepatomegaly (Chapter 11): Enlargement of the liver.

Howell-Jolly bodies (Chapter 4): Small remnants of the erythrocyte nucleus that occasionally remain after the nucleus undergoes division.

Hyaluronic acid (hyaluronan) (Chapter 15): Joint fluid.

Hyperadrenocorticism (Cushing's disease) (Chapter 11):: A disease characterized by an overproduction of cortisol caused by primary adrenal or pituitary disease.

Hyperbilirubinemia (Chapter 4): Increased bilirubin in the bloodstream.

Hypercalcemia (Chapter 8): High blood levels of calcium.

Hypercalcemia of malignancy (Chapter 8): An increase in blood calcium levels caused by specific types of cancer.

Hypercholesterolemia (Chapter 9): High blood cholesterol levels.

Hyperglycemia (Chapter 7): Increased blood glucose levels.

Hyperkalemia (Chapter 5): High blood potassium levels.

Hypernatremia (Chapter 8): Increased serum sodium concentration.

Hyperphosphotemia (Chapter 5): Increased blood phosphorus levels.

Hyperproteinemia (Chapter 9): High blood protein levels.

Hypersplenism (Chapter 4): A splenic disease in which the spleen removes excessive numbers of erythrocytes due to abnormal macrophage function.

Hypertension (Chapter 5): Increased blood pressure.

Hypoadrenocorticism (Addison's disease) (Chapter 11):: A decreased production of aldosterone and/or cortisol by the adrenal gland.

Hypoalbuminemia (Chapter 5): Low blood albumin levels.

Hypocalcemia (Chapter 8): Low blood calcium levels.

Hypochromia (Chapter 4): Red blood cells with decreased staining of their cytoplasm.

Hypoglycemia (Chapter 8): Low blood glucose levels.

Hypokalemia (Chapter 5): Low blood potassium levels.

Hyponatremia (Chapter 8): Low blood sodium levels.

Hypophosphatemia (Chapter 8): Decreased phosphorus concentration.

Hypoproteinemia (Chapter 5): Low blood protein levels.

Hyposthenuria (Chapter 5): Excretion of urine of unusually low specific gravity and limited concentration of solutes.

Hypotension (Chapter 14): Decreased blood pressure.

Iatrogenic hyperadrenocorticism (Chapter 11): A disease produced from long-term administration of exogenous steroids (i.e., prednisone), which can disrupt the normal negative feedback loop by causing suppression of ACTH section by the pituitary gland.

Icterus (Chapter 6): Jaundice.

Idiopathic disease (Chapter 11): A disease produced by an unknown cause.

Immune-mediated hemolytic anemia (Chapter 3): An immune disease wherein body antibodies attach to the membrane of normal erythrocytes inappropriately causing the body to destroy its red blood cells as if they were foreign bacteria, resulting in a regenerative anemia.

Immune response (Chapter 3): The body's cellular and chemical response to a foreign pathogen or material.

Immunoblasts (Chapter 4): Large lymphocytes with deeply basophilic cytoplasm and prominent nucleoli.

Immunoglobulin (Chapter 3): Proteins produced from lymphocytes that recognize specific foreign material.

Immunology (Chapter 3): The study of a complex cellular defense that recognizes foreign substances and infectious agents and mounts a reaction to destroy the foreign agent.

Induction (Chapter 6): A process whereby an enzyme is stimulated to be produced by an organ.

Insulin (Chapter 7): A pancreatic enzyme released in times of increasing blood sugar to stimulate the conversion of sugar into glycogen (liver) and fat.

Intrinsic pathway (Chapter 13): A stepwise chemical reaction that is involved in the formation of a fibrin clot.

Ischemia (Chapter 14): Lack of tissue oxygenation.

Jaundice (Chapter 5): A conditions that occurs when bilirubin, a waste product from red blood cell production, builds up in the tissue.

Juxtoglomerular cells (Chapter 5): Cells within the renal arterioles that secrete a hormone called renin to help maintain blood pressure.

Keratocytes (Chapter 4): Erythrocytes that have small blisters on their surface that occasionally rupture.

Ketones (acetone) (Chapter 7): A chemical compound that is produced in the severe, uncontrolled diabetic.

Köhler illumination (Chapter 1): The process of adjusting the condenser to produce the best focus of the illumination source.

Lactate (Chapter 14): A blood toxin that builds up secondary to altered energy production from glucose in the body due to decreased oxygen levels in the tissue.

Left-shift (Chapter 4): A release of immature neutrophils into the bloodstream.

Leukocytes (Chapter 1): White blood cells.

Leukocytosis (Chapter 1): An increased white blood cell count.

Leukopenia (Chapter 1): A decreased white blood cell count.

Leukophagia (Chapter 15): Body macrophages that have engulfed white blood cells.

Lipase (Chapter 7): A pancreatic enzyme that breaks down fat into smaller molecules so they can be absorbed by the intestine.

Lipemia (Chapter 5): A condition that suggests an increased white precipitate of fat or lipid in the serum.

Loops of Henle (Chapter 5): Specialized structures within the renal medulla that aid in the concentration of urine.

Lymph nodes (Chapter 3): Small round or oval structures within the subcutaneous tissue that function to filter extracellular fluid (lymph) for foreign material and produce white blood cells (specifically lymphocytes) that then produce antibodies in response to foreign infection.

Lymphangiectasia (Chapter 4): Dilated lymphatic vessels of the gastrointestinal tract.

Lymphatics (Chapter 3): Specialized thin-walled vessels that carry lymph throughout the body.

Lymphocyte (Chapter 3): A white blood cell responsible for producing acquired immunity to infection.

Lymphocytopoiesis (Chapter 3): Production of the lymphocyte from the bone marrow.

Lymphocytosis (Chapter 4): An increase in blood lymphocyte numbers.

Lympholysis (Chapter 4): Destruction of lymphocytes.

Lymphoma (Chapter 4): A cancer arising from the white blood cells of the body.

Lymphopenia (Chapter 4): Decreased numbers of circulating lymphocytes.

Macroplatelets (Chapter 2): Large platelets found in the blood.

Malabsorption (Chapter 7): The inability to absorb nutrients properly.

Malassezia (Chapter 15): A common yeast found in the ears and on the skin of patients.

Maldigestion (Chapter 7): The inability to digest food properly.

Mean cell hemoglobin concentration (MCHC) (Chapter 2):: The ratio of hemoglobin to red blood cell size.

Mean cell volume (MCV) (Chapter 2): A direct measurement of cell size, which is related to the magnitude of the disrupted electrical current as each cell passes through the instrument.

Mean corpuscular hemoglobin (MCH) (Chapter 2): The amount of hemoglobin present in the red blood cells.

Mean corpuscular hemoglobin concentration (MCHC) (Chapter 9): The average percent measurement of hemoglobin concentration in each red blood cell.

Megakaryopoiesis (Chapter 3): The production of platelets in the bone marrow.

Melena (Chapter 7): The presence of digested blood in the feces, as noted by a dark, tarry-looking stool.

Mesenchymal tumors (Chapter 15): Tumors that arise from the supportive tissues of the body.

Metabolic acidosis (Chapter 12): A condition that occurs when the blood pH decreases below 7.35 due to the buildup of toxins, decrease in glomerular filtration, and/or the loss of bicarbonate rich fluids.

Metarubricytes (Chapter 4): Nucleated red blood cells (nRBC).

Microangiopathy (Chapter 4): The formation of fibrin strands or small fibrin clots within capillaries, which is associated with disseminated intravascular coagulation.

Microcytic (Chapter 4): A red blood cell with decreased volume.

Mineralocorticoid (Chapter 11): A hormone released by the adrenal cortex to help reabsorb electrolytes from the kidneys.

Minimal clinical databases (Chapter 14): A set of clinical diagnostic tests run to evaluate an emergency or hospitalized patient.

Modified transudates (Chapter 15): A fluid obtained from a body cavity with a total protein between 2.5–3.5 mg/dL and a total cell count between 1000–5000 cell/μL.

Monocyte (Chapter 3): A large white blood cell whose primary function is to migrate to the tissues to become a macrophage, a tissue white blood cell that is involved in controlling chronic infectious diseases.

Mucopolysaccharidosis VI (Chapter 4): A rare inherited disease that is characterized by abnormal leukocytes.

Mycoplasma hemofelis and *Mycoplasma hemominutum* (Chapter 4): Two erythroparasites that attach to the surface of the erythrocyte.

Myoglobin (Chapter 9): A compound similar to hemoglobin that is responsible for carrying oxygen and removing carbon dioxide in the muscle tissue.

Myoglobinuria (Chapter 9): The presence of myoglobin in the urine.

Necrosis (Chapter 4): Tissue death.

Neoplasia (Chapter 6): Cancer.

Neutropenia (Chapter 3): A decreased neutrophil population.

Neutrophil (Chapter 3): The most common granulocyte in the peripheral blood of dogs, cats, humans, and horses.

Neutrophilia (Chapter 3): An increased neutrophil number.

Nitrous oxide (Chapter 13): A chemical released from endothelial cells to prevent clot formation.

Nonregenerative anemia (Chapter 4): An anemia with no evidence that the bone marrow can respond.

Norepinephrine (Chapter 11): A chemical neurotransmitter involved with the sympathetic nervous system.

Oncotic pressure (Chapter 5): The force exerted by albumin on the fluid component of the blood, pulling fluid from the tissue into the blood so that the large protein molecule can be moved through the vascular supply.

Packed cell volume (PCV) (Chapter 14): A clinical diagnostic test that evaluates the red blood cell column as compared to the entire column of blood and fluid in a hematocrit tube.

Pancreatic exocrine insufficiency (PEI) (Chapter 7):: A rare congenital or acquired disease of the acinar cells resulting in a lack of production of exocrine pancreatic enzymes.

Pancreatitis (Chapter 7): An inflammation or infection of the pancreas producing a leakage of lipase and amylase onto the organ surface.

Panhypoproteinemia (Chapter 9):: Abnormally small amounts of total protein in the circulating plasma.

Papilloma (Chapter 15): A benign tumor that arises from the squamous epithelial cells of the skin.

Parathyroid hormone (PTH) (Chapter 8): A hormone released by the parathyroid gland that increases the blood level of calcium by removing calcium from the bone.

Parfocal (Chapter 1): Having the focal points of a lens all in the same plane. This means that if the image is in focus at $10\times$, there should be little need to focus at the higher magnification objectives.

Pelger-Huët anomaly (Chapter 4): A genetic disease found in many breeds of dogs and occasional cats. In individuals affected with Pelger-Huët anomaly, all circulating neutrophils and eosinophils are hyposegmented and resemble band forms of these granulocytes.

Pellet (Chapter 9): The cellular sample of a fluid that has been separated by centrifugation.

Phagocytize (Chapter 3): A cell's ability to extend its cell wall around foreign material and cells and internalize the structures.

Pheochromocytoma (Chapter 11):: Cancer of the adrenal medulla.

Phosphorus (Chapter 8): A mineral integral in many cell functions, including bone formation, energy metabolism, muscle contraction, and acid/base balance.

Pituitary-dependent hyperadrenocorticism (PDH) (Chapter 11):: A form of hyperadrenocorticism caused by a pituitary tumor, which produces excessive amounts of ACTH and causes overstimulation of both adrenal glands resulting in constant production of cortisol.

Pituitary gland (Chapter 11): A small gland that sits at the base of the brain and produces releasing hormones for other endocrine glands of the body.

Poikilocytosis (Chapter 4): An indication that the red blood cells seen on review of a blood film have variable shapes.

Polychromatophilic red blood cells (Chapter 4):: Erythrocytes that are usually larger than normal erythrocytes, have a larger central pallor, have a blue hue when stained with Wright-Giemsa stain, and have a muddy blue hue when stained with Diff-Quik™.

Polycythemia (Chapter 4): The counterpoint to anemia; an increase in red blood cell count, Hct/PCV, and hemoglobin.

Polycythemia vera (Chapter 4): A neoplastic process that results in production of high numbers of red blood cells.

Polydipsia (Chapter 5): Increased thirst.

Polyphagia (Chapter 8): Increased appetite.

Polyuria (Chapter 5): Increased urination.

Poodle macrocytosis (Chapter 4): A genetic trait that results in a normal MCV higher than other dogs.

Porphyrin (Chapter 9): A heme pigment.

Portacaval shunt (Chapter 6): A small blood vessel, called a shunt, that can occur from the portal vein to the caudal vena cava producing a bypass of blood flow around the liver. In affected patients, blood toxins enter the general bloodstream producing severe neurological and systemic signs.

Portal venous system (Chapter 6): The large venous system carrying bacteria, nutrients, and toxins from the intestine into the liver.

Postparturient hypocalcemia (Chapter 10):: Eclampsia.

Postrenal azotemia (Chapter 5): A rise in kidney enzymes due to an obstruction of the bladder, which produces a retrograde backflow of urine to the kidneys.

Potassium (Chapter 5): An intracellular ion that helps produce electrical energy allowing skeletal and cardiac contraction muscle, depolarization of nerves, and other metabolic functions.

Prerenal azotemia (Chapter 5): A condition caused by decreased blood perfusion of the kidneys producing decreased glomerular filtration.

Prostaglandin I (Chapter 13): A chemical released from endothelial cells to prevent clot formation.

Protein-losing enteroopathy (Chapter 7): Low body albumin. Patients with malabsorption/maldigestion disease (e.g., inflammatory bowel disease, lymphangectasia, intestinal neoplasia) can have depletions in essential amino acids and proteins, producing hypoalbuminemia.

Protein-losing nephropathy (Chapter 5): A syndrome wherein increased body protein (albumin) is excreted in the urine.

Proteinuria (Chapter 5): The presence of protein (albumin) in the urine.

Prothrombin (Chapter 13): The inactivated form of thrombin.

Prothrombin time (PT) (Chapter 13): An assay that evaluates the extrinsic clotting pathway.

Pseudohyperkalemia (Chapter 8):: Non-pathologic conditions that produce a non–life-threatening or artifactual hyperkalemia, including chronic GI parasitism, specific breed variations, and marked thrombocytosis.

Pyuria (Chapter 9): Neutrophils in the urine.

Refractometer (Chapter 5): An instrument used to measure the concentration of urine.

Regenerative anemia (Chapter 4): An anemia with evidence that the bone marrow can respond by increased production of erythrocytes.

Renal azotemia (Chapter 5): A condition caused by a disease that primarily affects the kidneys and decreases medullary concentration.

Renal cortex (Chapter 5): The part of the kidney that is responsible for the filtration of toxins out of the blood, balancing of blood electrolytes, and control of blood pressure.

Renal medulla (Chapter 5): The part of the kidney that is responsible for the concentration of urine to prevent dehydration.

Renin (Chapter 5): A hormone secreted by juxtoglomerular cells of the kidney that activate angiotensin.

Renin-angiotensin system (Chapter 5): A system utilized by the kidneys to help maintain blood pressure.

Respiration (Chapter 14): A process whereby energy is produced from glucose in the presence of oxygen.

Respiratory acidosis (Chapter 12): A condition that occurs when the blood pH decreases below 7.35 due to the buildup of carbon dioxide from improper gas exchange in the lungs.

Reticulocytes (Chapter 1): Immature red blood cells released from the bone marrow at a less mature phase in response to body need. These cells maintain remnants of their internal structures and will stain differently under specific stains.

Reticulocytosis (Chapter 2): An increased number of immature red blood cells.

Ringworm (Chapter 15): A common fungal skin infection.

Romanowsky stain (Chapter 3): A stain used to evaluate blood smears.

Romanowsky stain (Diff-Quik™) (Chapter 1): A stain system that stains the components of a cell different colors depending on the structure's pH.

Sarcoptes (Chapter 15): A skin mite.

Schistocytes (Chapter 4): Small fragments of erythrocytes that are irregular in size and shape.

Sepsis (Chapter 4): Whole-body massive infection.

Siderocytes (Chapter 4): Erythrocytes with iron-containing basophilic inclusions.

Sodium (Chapter 8): The most abundant positively charged ion in the extracellular fluid that helps regulate electrical potential in the body.

Sodium/potassium balance (Chapter 11): The ratio of blood serum levels of sodium compared to potassium.

Spherocytes (Chapter 4): Small erythrocytes with no central pallor. Spherocytes are a hallmark of immune-mediated hemolytic anemia, but they also can be seen in small numbers in association with other types of erythrocyte damage.

Squamous cell carcinoma (Chapter 15): A malignant tumor of the squamous cells of the skin.

Standard deviation (Chapter 1): A measure of the variability or dispersion of a population, a data set, or a probability distribution.

Staphylococcus (Chapter 15): A common skin bacteria.

Stem cell (Chapter 3): Undifferentiated cells, from which individual cells will commit to a specific cell type.

Steroid hepatopathy (Chapter 11): A metabolic disease of the liver caused by increased chronic steroid-affecting liver tissue.

Stress leukogram (Chapter 5): Changes noted in a complete blood count when the patient is in a stressful environment.

Struvite crystals (Chapter 9): The most common crystal seen in companion animal urine.

Supernatant (Chapter 9): The fluid portion left after a sample (urine) is centrifuged.

Suppurative infection (Chapter 15): An infection, or inflammatory disease, that has the capability of forming pus (neutrophils).

Target cells (codocytes) (Chapter 4): Erythrocytes with a central area of hemoglobin within the area of central pallor forming a target appearance.

Thrombin (Chapter 13): An enzyme responsible for the formation of fibrin; also, the inappropriate formation of a clot in the blood vessel.

Thrombocytopenia (Chapter 1): A decreased platelet count.

Thrombocytosis (Chapter 1): An increased platelet count.

Thrombopoietin (Chapter 3): A hormone responsible for the production of platelets.

Total protein (TP) (Chapter 14): A measurement of the serum that evaluates the sum of blood albumin and globulin levels.

Toxic neutrophil (Chapter 4): A neutrophil that has increased cytoplasmic basophilia and a moth-eaten or foamy change to its cytoplasm.

Transitional cells (urothelial cells) (Chapter 9):: Cells that line the bladder wall, vary considerably in size, and have rounded edges and variable amounts of cytoplasm.

Transudates (Chapter 15): A fluid obtained from a body cavity with a total protein of <2.5 mg/dL and a total cell count of <1000 cell/μL.

Trigone (Chapter 5): A region in the neck of the bladder where the ureters enter.

Urine protein/creatinine ratio (Chapter 5): A clinical diagnostic that measures the amount of protein in the urine in comparison to the amount of creatinine.

Urine specific gravity (Chapter 5): The measure of concentration of the urine.

Ventroflexion of the neck (Chapter 5): A syndrome that occurs when the body's potassium is so low that the patient cannot lift its neck.

von Willebrand's disease (Chapter 13): Deficiencies in factors that allow the platelet to adhere to the subendothelial tissue.

Whole blood clotting time (Chapter 13): A clinical diagnostic measure of the time it takes for blood drawn into a serum tube to clot.

Zona fasciculata and Zona reticularis (Chapter 11): The inner regions of the adrenal cortex that produce a prednisone-like steroid called cortisol and small amounts of androgens (sex hormones).

Zona granulosa (Chapter 11): The outermost area of the adrenal cortex, which is responsible for producing a steroid hormone called aldosterone, also called a mineralocorticoid.

Index

Page references followed by a denote algorithms; those followed by b denote text boxes; those followed by c denote charts; those followed by f denote figures; those followed by t denote tables.

A

Acanthocytes, 45, 46f, 47–48, 47t, 56, 212t, 259
Acetolactate, 143–144
Acetone, 114, 116, 143
Acidosis
  causes of, 167–169, 168f, 171a, 230f
  definition, 259
  discussing importance of monitoring blood gas with client,
    173–174
  evaluation process, 170–173
    algorithm for, 171a
    step 1 (identity acidosis), 170
    step 2 (determine type of acidosis), 170
    step 3 (develop differential list), 173
    step 4 (treatment plan formulation), 172–173
  lactic, 167
  metabolic, 167–174, 168f, 170f
  respiratory, 168–173, 169f
Acquired immunity, 33
ACTH. *See* Adrenocorticotrophic hormone (ACTH)
ACTH stimulation test, 159–160
  in hyperadrenocorticism, 163
  in hypoadrenocorticism, 165
Activated partial thromboplastin time (aPTT), 180–182,
    181t, 182c, 191c, 259
Addisonian crisis, 152, 153, 157, 259
Addison's disease. *See* Hypoadrenocorticism
Adenocarcinoma, 202, 259
Adenoma, 202, 259
ADH (antidiuretic hormone), 141, 142f
Adipocytes, 202f
Adrenal cortex, 151, 259
Adrenal glands, 151–166
  anatomy, 151, 152f
    adrenal cortex, 151
    adrenal medulla, 151

function
  cortisol production, 152, 153f
  epinephrine production, 153, 155
  mineralocorticoid production, 152–153, 154f
hyperadrenocorticism (Cushing's disease), 155–164
  adrenal neoplasia, 156–157, 157f
  clinical signs of, 155, 155f
  diagnosis of, 157–162, 162f, 229f
  iatrogenic, 157
  monitoring, long-term, 162–164, 163f
  pituitary-dependent (PDH), 156, 156f
hypoadrenocorticism (Addison's), 164–166
  causes, 164
  diagnostic tests, 165–166, 166b
  primary, 164–165
  secondary, 165
pheochromocytoma, 166
Adrenal medulla, 151, 259
Adrenal-mineralocorticoid axis, 119
Adrenal-pituitary axis, 152
Adrenocorticotrophic hormone (ACTH)
  definition, 259
  stimulation of cortisol release by, 152, 153f
AG (anion gap), 172, 208t, 260
Agglutination of erythrocytes, 14, 59, 59f, 60f
Akita
  erythrocyte size, 53
  hyperkalemia in, 122
  potassium values in, 17
Alanine aminotransferase (ALT)
  definition, 259
  in hyperadrenocorticism, 159
  increased activity, 99
  low activity, 99
  normal values, 99c, 208t

Printed and bound by CPI Group (UK) Ltd, Croydon, CR0 4YY
21/08/2022
03142857-0001